A Rose to a Sick Friend

A Positive Way to Approach your Illness

Tessa Goldhawk

Gateway Books, Bath

First published in 1989
by Gateway Books
The Hollies, Wellow,
Bath, BA2 8QJ

© 1989 by Tessa Goldhawk

Cover design by Studio B, Bristol
Cartoons by Tony Weare
Set in 10½ on 12 Sabon by
Mathematical Composition Setters Ltd.
of Salisbury
Printed and bound by Billings
of Worcester

British Library Cataloguing in Publication Data:
Goldhawk, Tessa, *1954*–
    A rose to a sick friend: a positive way
    to approach your illness
    1. Man. Sickness. Personal adjustment
    I. Title
    362.1'

ISBN 0-946551-51-0

Contents

To my Mother and Father
and to all who care

Introduction

This book is not intended to be an original book of wisdom. I realise that many of the things I write in here, you will already know. But I write it because of my own long experience of being ill (I am, you could say, an expert in being ill!) and I know that during certain crises in our lives it is very useful to hear other people telling us the truths we already know in our hearts.

If you are lucky you may have friends who will gather round your sick bed and do this for you—reminding you that although you know something, you may not actually take any notice of it! If you are lucky, you may find help and insight coming from all sorts of unexpected quarters.

It may be, for many reasons, that during your illness you find yourself often alone. Consider this book a delicate red rose to a sick friend. Something you can turn to if you need it, which may, with any luck, give you a fresh understanding, some joy, maybe laughter, and hopefully comfort.

This is the book I've often wished I'd had to read in my darkest days of getting well.

Patient's Check List

1. Have I contacted my GP?
2. Do I like and trust my GP?
3. Have I had my symptoms diagnosed either by my GP or a specialist to my satisfaction?
4. Does the treatment offered suit me?
5. Are they prepared to accept my seeing an alternative practitioner?
6. Have I considered: Acupuncture, Bach Flower Remedies, Herbalism, Homeopathy or Osteopathy as a long term treatment of my illness?
7. Do I like and trust my Complementary Medicine practitioner?
8. Does the Complementary Medicine I have chosen suit me?
9. Can I contact my practitioner in emergencies?
10. If not, will they accept my going to my GP?
11. Do I want additional healing?
12. Have I been in touch with my local Federation of Healers, or a healer I know of personally?

If your answer to any of these questions is NO, and you feel unhappy about that, perhaps you should put this book down and get someone to help you to change your situation.

1

The Incredible Journey

There is a pattern to regaining health that is really very simple, though when we are caught up in the fear and pain of illness, it can seem hard to grasp. It goes like this:

Step One: First accept that you are ill. This does not mean giving in to the illness and dying of it. It means giving up the delusion that you can go on exactly as you did when you were well.

Step Two: Let go of the stress and worries which stop you accepting you are ill, and change your thoughts from "I can't afford to be ill because..." to "So, I'm ill, how can I help myself recover?"

Step Three: Encourage your mind to become interested in helping you recover, then it is less likely to fall into fear and panic (The perhaps I'll die...what will happen tomorrow...what's wrong, why does the pain HURT so?...perhaps my legs will drop off...).

Step Four: Consider that your illness has something to teach you. You can consider this either practically or more deeply. Practically: if you are going to lie there for a certain amount of time, you might as well make use of it. On a deeper level: nothing in life just happens to us. There are always events leading up to an illness which put us in danger of being ill: stress at work; emotional upsets; unspoken fears or angers.

Sometimes these dangers to our health seem to be events outside our control: sudden loss, for example. Sometimes these events are clearly to do with our own behaviour, attitudes and actions. Whether or not you can see a pattern leading to your illness, you have to admit it is now part of your life—maybe a most unexpected part.

Step Five: Accept you are living your own life (and having your own illness). You are not Mrs Jones who didn't get ill and who did what you did, or Mr Smith who died. The events you are experiencing now are your own teaching.

Step Six: Learn whatever you need to learn in order to get well.

This process of accepting, letting go, learning, growing, and then throwing off the illness may be one you only have to go through once, or, if you have a lot to learn, you may go through it—up and down—many times.

Don't be afraid. It is not difficult. It is not dangerous. While the thought of whatever darkness is disturbing you may seem terrifying now, it is nothing you cannot handle. Each one of us is born on this planet as a soul wanting to grow further towards the Divine Light. We are never given more than we can handle on the journey towards greater self-understanding and perfection.

Each suffering we undergo may seem at the time to weaken our bodies, but it is always an opportunity for us to strengthen our soul; our inner centre; our wisdom and our contact with the Source. (Whatever that is for each of us.) Illness is one of the ways we are given to learn about ourselves, and to grow. If we let it, it can be a moving and inspiring journey—so much so that at the end of weeks or months of pain and disease, we hear ourselves saying: "I'm glad I went through that: it has changed me and I'm grateful for the change".

It is extraordinary that something rife with depression and despair, with pain and terror, can lift our spirits higher, but it can. Illness is a wonderful opportunity!

Through this book I am going to embark on this incredible journey with you. At the moment you are no doubt feeling you would happily give away all the pain and discomfort you have,

rather than journey through it. Too bad you can't.
Good luck and many blessings to you.

2

Pain

DON'T PANIC

These words were made famous in a book called *The Hitchhiker's Guide to the Galaxy.* "Don't Panic" the guide book said, when you find yourself adrift in the vastness of space, no matter what strange planet or spaceship or time warp you find yourself in. These words apply to you now. You have also found yourself suddenly in the middle of a vast unknown. Of course you are panicking: You're upset, ready to believe the worst. The equilibrium of your life is upset and, hardest of all, you don't know how to get the balance back again.

When you are ill it's no good anyone telling you to be sensible, or to pull yourself together. Though you might agree with them intellectually, nothing can counter the blind horror and fear you feel when you are suddenly caught up in pain and illness. But I know there is a small part of you that raised a little smile when you read those first words, and no matter how awful you feel, if you hold this book still for one minute, and breathe as deeply as you can, and breathe deeply again, you will immediately know that the part of you which watches everything—including your own suffering—is still there within you now.

At this moment that is all you need to know. Keep conscious of your breathing as you continue to read. Breathe as deeply and as calmly as possible, and keep listening to your breath going in and out, in and out.

Breath is life. You are breathing and you are alive. Let all the rest of your world fall away from you for a minute. The events which brought you to this place, your worries about the future.... let them move apart from you like a dull grey mist, present all around you, but just that little bit apart from you. And in the small space you can make, keep your attention on your calm and deep breathing.

Don't worry if you find yourself feeling tearful or frustrated or any other strong feelings. Let those feelings be there too, fading away gently to be part of the grey mist around you.

Continue to pay attention to these words and your breath for just a moment longer. This exercise is about giving yourself exactly the space you need, right now, to find the fine person who still exists at your centre. In the middle of the thick·grey mist, there's just a little chink of light, and a bright clear ray of sun.

Let me say straight away: you are not being punished by being ill. This is a common feeling, along with the feeling that it is completely unjust and unfair that it should happen to you. Both of these reactions are OK, but neither of them are accurate.

You may well be ill as a result of events for which you are responsible (such as overworking yourself), but none of us is able to be more than human. We will all do things that lead us to a point in life, at some time or other, like the one you find yourself in now.

When we are ill everyone around us suddenly seems so lucky, and so healthy in comparison, so it is important to remember that this is only a point in your life, and nearly everyone will go through, or has been through a terrible point in their lives too.

"Welcome to the human race" was one of the nice things one of my visitors to my sick bed said to me.

WELCOME TO THE HUMAN RACE

Perhaps as soon as you started to breathe more deeply you became aware of how tightly you were holding onto yourself. As if in fear that letting go of any part of your body would result in more pain, more shock, more bleeding and so on. It may be you feel that letting go of any part of yourself will make you feel dizzy or sick, or put extra pressure on a hurt place you are protecting, and you will be 'out of control'.

Let me give you a picture: A man is using a saw and suddenly he cuts his arm badly. He withdraws the arm quickly, holds his breath and his mind starts racing, his body starts pumping adrenaline, his muscles tighten—everything, in fact, gets set for 'fight or flight'. That is, taking us at our basic animal level, a serious injury means we are either being attacked and need to defend ourselves, or we need to run for help.

Now let's say this man runs and finds someone to help him, and the wound is patched up. His body starts to wind down when suddenly the potential danger of his situation (he could have bled to death) hits him, and he starts to feel dizzy and sick. He could also feel upset or angry at himself, but this man is afraid of feeling those very natural feelings. He is afraid of feeling dizzy and sick. He therefore repeats the old pattern *which worked for him before*: he holds his breath, tightens his muscles, his mind starts racing, his body pumping adrenaline. But this time the emergency is over, and he has nothing external to fight, nowhere to run to. Therefore his body reactions are *not appropriate to the situation*.

Among all the animals, only humans can keep on stimulating inappropriate body reactions after the time has passed—because of the very great power of our conscious and unconscious mind.

What this man needs to do—as any animal would do—is to lie down, rest, calm and deepen his breathing, thus allowing his heart rate to lessen and his blood to flow more evenly, allowing his muscles to stop contracting, and thus giving the nerve fibres opportunity to feed more appropriate messages to the brain and central nervous system, so that his body can get on with the next step: the process of repairing and healing.

By relaxing and breathing calmly you cannot make your illness worse, you can only aid your body to set about the business of making yourself better. If you allow the whole of your lungs (right from the middle of your back, under your. armpits, to the area right under your collar bones) gently to fill with air; this gives your body more oxygen, which gives you energy, and energy is what your body needs to heal itself.

Of course this is easier understood intellectually than done. For one thing, if the man in our story had lain down, he would *at first* have felt more dizzy and sick, and once the pain-killing effect of the adrenaline wore off, his nerve fibres would relay the true extent of the pain to his brain, so of course he would experience the pain as worsening.

DON'T BE AFRAID OF PAIN

If it helps, take pain killers. I am not advocating lying there suffering for the sake of suffering. Nor is it a good idea to concentrate on your pain for too long. But do not be afraid of pain—it is simply your body telling you all is not well. Do not be afraid of pain because the body, your body, is an incredible creation, and there are many things that you, and others can do, to heal and ease your pain.

Many creative acts are born of pain. Our own lives began with our mother's pain. Getting to know and love ourselves will only come through pain. For some reason best known to the Universal Plan of things, this is the nature of our lives as human beings, just as much as gravity is in the nature of energetic force on this planet.

Included in this book are some ways we can approach our pain, and stimulate our own self-healing. You can turn now to these on pages 125 to 134 or wait and read on, and use one or all of them later when you feel like it.

> Your pain is the breaking of the shell that encloses your understanding.
> Even as the stone of the fruit must break, that its heart may stand in the sun, so must you know pain.
>
> (Kahlil Gibran)

I know, because I have experienced many times, pain going on and on and on. I know tossing in a bed which seems to grow harder and more uncomfortable to hip bones that ache, and shoulders which are sore.

I know pains like knives which seem to slice through your insides. Pains that are hot and itching, and seem so angry and insistent, you want to scream. I know headaches where the huge throb of a dark weight inside your head is like a stone mashing your brains. Nausea and sickness where you feel like a limp worm leaking from both ends.

And there is no doubt: pain hurts!

PAIN HURTS

Sometimes it helps to remind yourself that 'all pain must pass', including the one you are experiencing now. Cheer yourself up by thinking back to a pain or illness you had in the past, and realise it is now over.

The important thing is to try not to hurry (or get desperate because it's taking so l o n g), but to breathe deeply and listen to your quiet inner self.

Take one minute, one hour, one day at a time. You have transferred from *well* mode, on this stranger inner spaceship, to *ill* mode. Time in ill mode is a completely different experience. Allow the hours to pass.

3

Worries and Anxieties

Doctor: Well now, is your cough better this morning?
Patient: It should be. I've been practising all night.

As soon as we begin any illness, all the resources of our body
gather together to try and make us well. Often the healing
process requires us to stop moving, or even to cut down our
activities to the absolute minimum—in other words to sleep.
Thus pain and tiredness and sickness are our body's very
logical way of literally 'cutting out' the engines, so that healing
can take place.

It may be that we go onto a light diet, or even to want only
liquids, so that our stomach and digestive organs have less
work to do. Although many people panic about loss of
appetite, in the short term it makes absolute sense to the body.
Your main concern at this stage is to cut down the one pressure
you can add to your already weak system: worry and anxiety.
If it makes you anxious not to eat, even though you have lost
your appetite, then eat. If it makes you feel terrible to eat if you
are not hungry, don't eat. (Though drink lots of liquids, but
not tea and coffee).

The whole subject of what to eat (or not eat) while ill is
important, but not within the scope of this book. In the
suggestions for further reading at the back, I have listed some
of the many good books which deal with diet. (The only thing I

would say now is the closer the food is to being raw, 'alive' and unadulterated, the more goodness it can offer you).

Worry and anxiety come hand in hand with illness. If you remember the man who cut himself with the saw—it was part of the adrenaline 'emergency' reaction that his mind started racing. As soon as we are out of balance our mind sways this way and that, dashing all our fears and terrors about in our head like nuts in a blender.

Remember—being vulnerable and prone to worry and fearfulness are symptoms of illness. Try not to make things worse by criticising yourself for this state.

I know—you know—that normally you are a perfectly capable human being. You have lived your life so far, and you will do so again. But right now you need to accept some assistance.

> There is no summer without the winter
> no blossom without the seed
> we are all born on this earth
> not just to give, but to receive.
>
> (Anon)

The luckiest thing any ill person can have is someone they can trust enough with whom to share their worries. Perhaps you have more than one person, in which case you can even share out your worries a little. But even if you feel you have no one, be sure to express your fears to someone. The ward orderly in the hospital, or the neighbour who comes around to complain about your rubbish—anyone could turn out to have a sympathetic ear just for the moment you need them. At times it is vital to say things OUT LOUD. You know—and I know—that some of your worries are unnecessary, but if you express them (even briefly) they will float off into the Universe. Keep them to yourself and they will add to the rattle of nuts in your brain.

Perhaps you are the sort of person who doesn't like asking for help, who hates having to show any weakness. Look at it this way: Now is a golden opportunity for you to practise something you are not good at. Think about this: when you consider all the people on the planet Earth, is there anyone alive who does not deserve to be cared for when they are in a state of terrible pain and sickness?

Perhaps you can think of one or two—Hitler for example —whom you would find it hard in your heart to feel like helping. But all the rest—of course they are worthy of care and love! And you? Why are you any different?

You live in a Universe supported by love. This may be hard for you to believe right now. You may point to thousands of reasons why it doesn't feel true to you. All I can say is that if we meditate or pray—as long as we open in trust—the sense of being loved and supported is there. And this love is like air—it doesn't judge who breathes it, it just is. No matter what we have done, no matter how angry or unworthy we feel, the love doesn't make those sort of judgements. It just loves.

> Come
> Come wherever you are,
> Wanderer, worshipper,
> lover of learning
> it doesn't matter.
> Ours it not a caravan of despair.
> Come,
> even if you have broken
> your vows a thousand times,
> Come, come yet again.
> Come.
>
> (Mevlana Jelaluddin Rumi. 17th Cent. Sufi)

If God, or the Universe, can love you so completely, can you not begin to love yourself in this way? Ask for help if you need it. Trust that help will come. It may not be in the form you had in mind, nor offered in the manner you would have chosen, but help will come, if you will only accept it.

Children

If you have children (or dependents), particularly if they are used to depending solely on you for care, you will already have had to ask for help by the time you come to pick up this book.

No one who is not a parent can really understand the huge amount of guilt we feel for our children when we are not well. Not only are we unable to provide all the material things—

food we know they especially like, cooked the 'right way', discovered through long experience, for example—but we hardly have the energy to give them any affection, let alone all the comfort we feel they need, or the games they want to play.

In my experience children are always more grown up in an emergency than we ever give them credit for. They not only prove they can look after themselves, they also take care 'not to worry' their parents, and often go out of their way to give love, and presents. They, being still in touch with their hearts, know what love is about far better than we do.

It will do them a great deal of good to be able to give back something to you, in return for the years of care you've shown them. Let them have the chance to do so. See it this way: You are now teaching them about compassion. No child's education is complete without learning about this valuable aspect of human nature, and being encouraged to express it!

When we worry, as we inevitably do, about 'our poor child, she'll be so upset. She'll be worried, and anxious, lost, all alone...' we are not seeing what is really happening for our child. What we are doing is projecting our version of events onto her. When we are ill our own personal inner child rises up and becomes very strong. By this I mean: if you consider that we grow from a child to an adult bit by bit, year by year, layer by layer, we never lose the basic childish self with which we began life, we just add to and modify that self as we gain in experience and, perhaps, wisdom.

This inner child expresses us at our most fundamental level, and is totally different from the outer children sharing your life. When you worry that your child is 'anxious, lost, all alone' it's worth stopping for a minute and asking yourself: "Is that my child, or my own inner child I'm describing?"

Maybe we have just described our own state perfectly, while little Jack or Jill might feel quite differently. Perhaps the neighbour, friend or relative looking after them is letting them watch the TV programme you don't approve of, or giving them treats, or teaching them new games, or any number of things which seem new and exciting to a child. Until they are much older, children do not have an expectation of how things should be, as we do. They quickly adapt to a new order of things. Ironically the only thing which *will* really worry a child is if YOU seem worried and upset.

Looked at this way we are lucky to have children because we are forced, for at least a little of the day, to act with them as if 'everything is fine', which, of course, it is.

> You are a child of the Universe, no less than the trees or the stars, you have a right to be here. And whether or not it is clear to you, no doubt the Universe is unfolding as it should.
> (*Desiderata*)

Children do require energy, however, particularly if you feel responsible for them. And if you can arrange, in the early stages of an illness, for them to go and stay with someone else—DO. Perhaps someone quite unexpected will offer. Take them up. Don't worry: you owe them nothing. In the future you may be given ample opportunity to pay them back in some way, but if not, *they will be paid back*.

One of the basic laws of this Universe is that any giving we do comes back to us, and by giving they are only ensuring that when their time comes to need help, they will receive it. I am not, of course, saying don't be thankful.

> Your children are not your children.
> They are the sons and daughters of life's longing for itself
> They come through you but not from you
> And though they are with you yet they belong not to you.
>
> You may give them your love but not your thoughts
> For they have their own thoughts.
> You may house their bodies, but not their souls,
> For their souls dwell in the house of tomorrow,
> Which you cannot visit, nor even in your dreams.
> You may strive to be like them, but seek not to make them
>   like you
> For life goes not backward nor tarries with yesterday.
> You are the bows from which your children as living arrows
>   are sent forth.
> (Kahlil Gibran)

Give away your child to life—his or her life. You can't protect them from an ill parent—it has already happened! Your inner child is the one who most needs your love and concern. You are not being selfish—you are setting your children an example in how to heal themselves.

Money

If you are a wage earner, particularly if you are self-employed, or committed to your work, having to stop and allow yourself to be ill seems almost impossible. The best thought I can offer is this: getting up too soon is a FALSE ECONOMY.

My own behaviour was a good example of this. Being self-employed I only earned money if I worked. Further I was very committed to my clients and didn't want to let them down. Very soon after my initial illness I convinced myself I was well enough and went back to work. I ignored all the warning signs (feeling pain and tiredness) until my body forced me to stop by collapsing. Because of the extra stress I put on my already weak body I had eventually to spend eight months regaining my health. If I had been wise and had waited, I firmly believe I could have halved my recovery time.

I use myself as an example, because I do not want you to think I am being superior and wise. You may, like me, have to learn your limits yourself by making exactly the same mistakes. As I see it, part of the process of getting well is learning what we can and cannot do, and looking at why it all matters so much to us anyway.

Of course you do not want to be penniless, and no doubt you cannot afford to be. But finally it all boils down to a simple question: which is more important to you, your health or money? Are the standards of living you wish to maintain worth any price? Do the goals you wish to pursue have to be gained right away? Only you can decide. But be sure that you don't settle on an equation that gives you a short term gain which you will inevitably have to to pay back—with high interest-—later.

Perhaps there are certain factors that you are not taking into account: have you thought about the advantages of having a strong body, a greater inner strength? A deeper approach to life? Maybe there is something in all your sums you are missing out? Maybe giving yourself attention now will greatly increase your success later. Maybe, maybe not.

> Once there was a young boy who was hungry. By the roadside he found a nut. He held the nut in his hand with great joy—now he had something to eat! It was not a large nut, but he gripped it tightly, because he knew it was the difference between life and death to him, and he set off down the road again, anxiously looking for a stone to crack the nut open.   ·
>
> He was so busy looking for a stone that he hardly noticed a stranger who was sat by the side of the road, in the shade of a small tree. The stranger, seeing the boy looked hungry, broke off a large chunk of the loaf of bread he was eating, and offered this, along with a large juicy apple.
>
> Astonished, the boy put out his hand to receive the food, but his fingers were still gripped tightly over the nut, and he could not let go and open his hand. The stranger, seeing the boy raise what he thought was a fist, grabbed his food to him, bound up on his horse, and disappeared.
>
> (Ancient Hebrew Tale)

One approach that might make things easier is this: consider how often, when you were working, you longed to have a day or two just doing what you liked. What about the books you longed to read? The things you longed to make?

Consider how you envied someone who had the time to think, simply to sit and look. And above all, time to get to know himself, and take stock of his life.

When I was ill I surveyed my life event by event, from its beginning to the present day. To my surprise I realised I had never done this, and in doing it I felt somehow whole, complete. It was a truly wonderful thing to do.

If you are reading this with your mind still caught up in your work, I suspect you will feel impatient, feel that I don't understand, sigh to yourself: how could I ever take the time to do that just now!

What I am saying is that you can either spend your illness

fretting that you are not well, trying to drive yourself way beyond your physical capacity, or you can accept that you are ill and get something out of it.

If it helps, set a time limit (which you can review at a later date). Say, for example: for the next two weeks I will concentrate on myself. You have a right to give your health some of the attention you put into your work. Your body is ill and it is asking you for help. You can try to ignore your own cries, if you like, but do you really want to?

If a small child suddenly became ill, and it was up to you, no matter where·you were—on a bus, in the middle of the night, at work—you would surely *stop everything* and help her. Do you not deserve the same?

4

Blocks to Regaining Health

In order to become well, we have to let ourselves be ill. This is simply a matter of accepting the ingredients we have lain out in front of us in order to make the cake. We do not try to make a cherry cake if we have sultanas. We cannot make a disease of the nervous system better by worrying about it, any more than we can heal a cut knee by constantly bending our leg.

We can see the cut knee has to be rested to heal, and the same relentless logic applies to a more complex disease. But once we have accepted that we are ill, and agreed we need to let ourselves rest, we still have to keep to our decision. It's easy enough when you are flat out with exhaustion, but the problem comes the moment you feel a spark of life. As soon as the brain finds enough spare energy to start questioning, you can easily start piling up the pressures to be up and about.

Why, when we know what we need, do we give ourselves such a hard time? These are a few reasons I can think of; maybe one of them applies to you.

1. The Fear of being a burden

During our childhood we were proud of each step we took which made us less dependent on our parents. Even though we needed their love and support, we were preoccupied with our dependence and the achievements which marked us 'adult'.

Independence is precious to most of us, and becoming ill

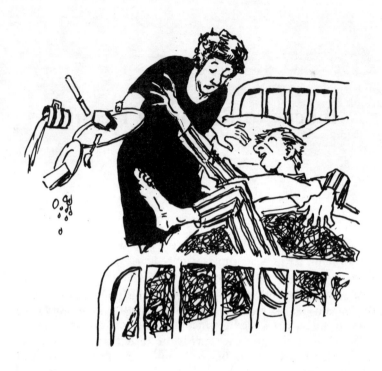

suddenly faces us with being right back in the early days of our childhood—needing to be fed and cared for, needing help.

Most of us feel a kind of shame at being in this situation, a wish to tell people 'I'm not normally like this'. At the same time we feel welling up in us a deep longing to be able to give in, and momentarily to be totally dependent on someone else.

No sooner have we fallen asleep in our warm bed, safe in the knowledge we are being looked after, than one of the voices in our head wakes us up with 'You must not be a burden. So and so has too much on her plate to worry about you'. And a horrible picture of ourselves emerges—as one big sack of troubles, that has to be carried on the back of someone else who is already carrying too many of their own sacks of troubles.

2. The Fear of being a failure

At school or at work, in our culture the emphasis is put on achievement. Success is counted by the things we do. Very few of us have the self-confidence to say 'I'm a nice person and that's achievement enough' although we could probably all think of someone else we could say that about.

In a world where everyone seems to be heading towards a winning post, being ill feels very much like being a failure. If we are one of the defective machines that do not seem to patch up quickly, that go on being ill despite immediate help, we can easily feel somehow we are not good enough.

With the pressure on the NHS to turn people out of beds as quickly as possible, I have sometimes felt even in hospital which should be the seat of caring, that getting well is a competition. Being told "Most people are back at work in two weeks" can set unrealistic expectations, which are bound to make us feel bad if we don't 'match up'.

While some people respond well to a challenge, many don't, and most of us need to balance the 'challenge' we set ourselves, with love and sympathy, whether we meet it or not.

3. The desire to be strong/nurturing

After we have reached adulthood we tend to take on certain roles in life. If we have partners or families, or people we work or hang around with, we tend to slot into being a certain way, not so much by choice, but more by small adaptations to external stimulae, until we roughly fit into the shape available to us. We then grow used to this shape.

Often we have one particular version of ourselves we like and are proud of. Perhaps it is that we are strong—that other people rely on us; that we are able to keep going when others tire. Perhaps we gain a feeling of pride through the things we have achieved because of our strength. Perhaps we gain a sense of self-respect from other people's admiring words and glances, from feeling we are 'better' than someone else we know. In the same way we may see ourselves as someone who cares about others, someone people can turn to. If we are a nurturer, any number of people will come to rely on us, and that may make us feel needed, and therefore loved and important.

When we are ill we can no longer fulfil our image of ourselves. Not only do we feel we have (and may really have) lost the love and respect we gained by being our old selves, we also feel that we have lost our very selves—our identity. If it is my identity to be strong, and I'm now ill in bed, I am not myself—I am unknown, a no one. This feeling is extremely scary, and it adds to the desperate urge most of us feel to regain our health as quickly as possible so things can be 'back to normal'.

4. The fear of loss of control

Another aspect of being an adult is being able to have at least some control over the way life is for us. Life itself is full of so many uncontrollables—from the weather to other people's love (or lack of it) for us—that we tend to build for ourselves at least some things we can rely on.

In this way our personal routines evolve—and they are no bad thing. There is a lot of emphasis in this Aquarian Age on 'going with the flow', on letting things 'happen themselves', but the danger is that unless we have a very strong centre and sense of purpose, we can find ourselves tossed about like leaves in the wind, never quite doing what we would have liked to have done.

Routines also have their negative side: by reducing our world to as few known variables as possible, we can fool ourselves into believing we are actually in control of life, instead of seeing our routines for what they are: useful frameworks which allow us to do what we set out to do.

If we do believe we are in control of our lives, a sudden event such as illness, a relationship splitting up, accident, death, or unemployment, can give us such an enormous shock it feels very hard to recover. Suddenly we are faced with our own smallness and vulnerability. For many of us feeling this is just too unbearable, and we search desperately for ways to feel we are back in control.

This search is by no means a bad thing, it is a drive which

helps us bounce back after sudden loss, and which can lead us up all sorts of creative avenues. But there are times, and illness is one of them, when we need to let ourselves be out of control for just a little while. Times when we have to hand over control to other people. Actually, once we let it happen it can be an enormous relief to take our position in the wings of the stage, and to realise *life goes on*, whether or not we pull the strings.

With any luck we'll be able to see some of the areas where we have controlled more than we needed to. Perhaps, for instance, we are forced to accept our partner (or child) being capable and loving when we believed he was incapable without our support. But it is a difficult step for most of us to allow things to be 'out of our hands', and it takes us some time to adjust to the pleasures of it. The nature of illness though, is that we aren't in control (at least not the way we imagined it). If we were, we would be well; we would never have got ill in the first place.

5. The fear of being loved for too long

When we were babies we were loved simply because we were babies. Our very eyes and fingers, our snuffles and our smiles were adorable to people who looked at us. But as we grew we began to understand the message that we received love if we deserved it, and anger if we didn't. Even the most perfect of parents will inevitably give her child this message—for no human being can provide the constant love of the Divine, nor are they meant to.

Gradually, in among the pleasures of being loved, creeps a feeling of guilt about having too much love—or rather of wanting too much love when our mother or father does not want to (or cannot) give it.

As a mother I know this is unavoidable: there are times (such as bedtimes) when I decide to finish loving and get on with something else. Especially because of my own inability to give love—or to stand the giving and receiving of any more than a certain amount of love—I know that I have sometimes cut my son off from my love, when he might have wished for more.

When we are ill, and receiving attention from others, we find that worries can arise about accepting help and concern, which we often push away, or fret about, because of our own fear of receiving love. Allowing ourselves to be looked after, and wholeheartedly receiving the care we are offered—really accepting it and appreciating it—are things that may take a great deal of learning. *But they are worth learning.*

Considered from the point of view of the person doing the caring: it is far nicer to be appreciated and thanked for our help, than to have to look after someone who is always trying (and failing) to look after themselves; who won't rest properly and so 'wastes' all the time we've put into caring for them, who doesn't appreciate our cooking or way of doing things, and who always seems to be fretful and bristling.

People are, it's true, sometimes wary of being taken advantage of, and if we really begin to enjoy being loved and cared for, we may hit the 'needy nerve' of our carers, who feel there is a limit to how much love anyone should be given. Sometimes there is not a big distinction between the carer (who is supposed to be well) and the cared for (who is ill), and if the carer is in need of help themselves, their limits may be quite frail.

There is a general disapproval in our puritan society of someone having a good time being ill. In some ancient tribes ill people are put in their beds outside the huts, so that passers-by can sympathise, or sit with them for a moment, and give them advice and attention. This might not suit those of us who like to 'hole up and lick our own wounds', but it does give the ill person permission to be in need of attention and care.

I also give you permission to have as much care and love as you need—however endless, huge and ravenous the need may seem. Do you give yourself the same permission? Whether you have people around you or not, there are two endless sources of love ready and waiting: one is you, and the other is within you.

Being able to be thankful is such an art. It is not so easy as we think. Life is immaculate and so has to be it's appreciation: immaculate.

(Maharaji)

There is one thing that stands out in all the examples I have just given: they all involve images of ourselves *as reflected in other people's eyes*. They may be fears about what people will think of us, or fears about not being able to project our self-image to others. Here we are, lying in our sick bed, bleeding, or coughing or hurting and sweating, and we are still worried about our self-image!

We are still living out our old connections to the outside world, even though it doesn't exist any more. Surely this tells us something about the way we relate to (or 'live in') ourselves?

If we draw some circles we can begin to see what it looks like:

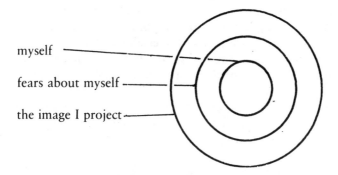

myself ——————

fears about myself ————

the image I project ————

The outer ring is the image I project to others. The way I hope or intend them to see me. For example I may feel sad, but when someone asks me how I am, I smile and say: 'I'm fine'. I try to project a nonchalant air. However it may be I don't project quite as well as I intended, and people are able to see through to my second layer, despite my efforts.

The second layer consists of my fears, my anxieties, and my distorted emotions (for example anger, which is directed at something quite different to the source that sparked it off, such as kicking the cat when I've had a bad day with my boss). This middle layer is the part of me rushing round trying to *cover-up* any of my emotions or experiences which I think are unacceptable.

The inner layer is my basic unadulterated self. The way I really feel and think when I am honest with myself. It is not a fixed thing—it changes from moment to moment, but we can know when we are 'there', when we are in touch with ourselves, because it feels 'right'. (And of course my diagram is not the way it actually is, but only my attempt to describe it, so we can have a picture.)

The circles of the drawing I have made, make the inner circle appear to be protected by the outer ones, but it is more accurate to see the outer layer (our projected image) as a semi-transparent sheet, which allows the two inner layers to show through, brightly in some places, dimly in others.

Often we are so involved in putting our attention onto the outer layer, however, that we forget about the other layers. And the inner self—the part of us everything comes from in the first place, the energy source for everything else—can grow gradually masked and distorted by the other two layers. Not just masked to other people, but *much more importantly* masked to ourselves.

This is known as being out of touch with our centre. In the fullness of everyday life it is very easy—even for those of us who know our centres well—to lose touch with ourselves. This is why many people meditate.

But now you are ill you are lucky enough to be at one of the rare points of your life where you have been stripped down to your bare essentials. When you recover, no doubt you will be back to your old tricks, but right now, fortunately for you, it is very hard for you to be so.

Why not take a deep breath and take a look at this new possibility? This is your chance to make up for any of the moments you missed; here you are, waiting to know yourself.

HELLO ME

To think about oneself is terrifying.
But it is the only honest thing:
to think about myself as I am, my
ugly features, my beautiful features,
and wonder at them. What other solid beginning can I have,
what to make progress from except myself?

(Mary Haskell)

Quiz for Sick Persons

Take a look at these questions, try to be honest with yourself, and if possible write down what you feel about each. Set aside at least half an hour, get pen and paper, and answer the following:

1. Who am I?
2. What do I believe in?
3. What do I fear?
4. What do I most admire about myself?
5. What do I love about myself?
6. What do I most doubt in myself?
7. What do I want?
8. What do I need?
9. What don't I need?
10. Why am I ill?

If you found answering these questions helpful, have you thought of keeping a notebook/journal to write down similar thoughts as they occur to you (just for yourself!)?

How to Deal with Visitors When Ill

1. When asked "How are you feeling?" always reply "Much better thank you", though if you are feeling worse , say it in a very weak voice.

2. On no account talk to visitors, or try to entertain them. This can be avoided by:
   a) mumbling incoherently.
   b) asking them a leading question about their favourite topic of conversation.
   c) keeping a thermometer handy and sticking it in your mouth whenever necessary.

3. Make a gigantic list of jobs so that anyone asking "Can I do anything to help?" can be given a job immediately. Even changing the water in the flowers will make them feel good, but if you want to help them feel really virtuous, give them a pot or sick bowl to slop out.

4. Leave clear evidence of doctor's visits: pills, prescriptions and so forth on display for all those people who want to tell you you should really be in Hospital. Also leave an article about cuts in Hospital beds slung casually on top of your bedside reading.

5. Leave your pills, Bach Flower remedies, Homeopathic remedies, Acupuncture moxxa etc. out in full view. Nothing pleases a visitor more than discussing the course of treatment you have chosen, and suggesting you might be better off trying something else.

6. Never discuss your symptoms with a visitor, unless you want to hear all about their last six illnesses, all of which will be more gruesome than yours.

7. If you are up when a visitor calls, get back into bed IMMEDIATELY. Once they think you are off the critical list they will stop coming and you never know when you might want that shopping done, baby minding, meal cooking etc.

8. Getting rid of a visitor:
   a) Close your eyes and breathe deeply
   b) Send them out shopping
   c) Close your eyes and snore loudly

If you do not want to see them at all—but you know they have travelled miles to see you etc, make sure you begin your greeting to them:

"It's so nice of you to come, unfortunately I have to have my enema in a minute."

5

The Miracle Pill

When we are ill the one thing we long for—when we are not longing to give up and die—is to be well. This is a good longing, and we can use this longing to help ourselves. For example when I was ill I used to repeat to myself, over and over:

"Every cell in my body is vibrating health
I am healing myself."

In this way I used the longing to help encourage myself to keep going in the right direction.

But the trouble with this longing to be well is that sometimes it can become so strong, so fierce that we try to head for it at 90 miles an hour, ignoring everything on the way.

The idea that attracts us most is: the Miracle Pill. Somewhere there must be something we can take (or do) which will make us well IMMEDIATELY. If only we could find it, all our problems would be over! But the point is that, unless you are very lucky, THERE IS NO MIRACLE CURE.

I know people who, for example, took the right homeopathic remedy and were well within a few weeks. I personally experienced having a long-term throat problem cured instantly by a faith healer. But—and this is a big but—for the majority of ills, cure is a more lengthy process.

We have to be careful not to be like the farmer who was so anxious to help his corn grow that he went out and tugged at the shoots. We may have the longing to get well in mind each day, but we have to allow sufficient time for our longing to come to fruition. If we 'tug at our shoots': worry, chop and change our medicines, keep trying to act well before we are, we may in the long run hinder our recovery, not help it.

In moments of doubt and panic we need to remind ourselves that our *frame of mind* is one of the most important aspects of our cure. It is also true that our 'frame of being' is equally important.

In order to reach our better state of health we have certain stages to go through. For some of us they will be few and we will get well quickly. If not we will take more time. If we spend our energy in trying to avoid going through those stages, we will take yet more time to get well.

To learn whatever you need to learn in order to get well may seem to be an arduous process, and the Miracle Pill may seem an easier way out. It is true, for instance, that many of us would choose to deaden our pain—even if this never cured it—rather than look at it.

But the point is this: If we learn a truth about ourselves we do not need to make the same mistake and learn the same truth ever again—and the learning adds to our fullness as human beings: in other words, we grow.

If we grow, *the whole of the rest of our lives* is transformed by the fact of our growth. We may get to places or have experiences that we never could have achieved without growing. We may find that knowing ourselves just that bit better helps our judgement in the subtlest of ways, ways we could not have conceived of.

> What the caterpillar calls the end of his life The sage calls a butterfly.
>
> (Richard Bach: *Illusions.*)

Time is never wasted if we keep in touch with ourselves and our centre/the Source. If we choose medicine A and it does not get us well as quickly as medicine B, who is to say that is a bad thing? Maybe we really need the extra time to be with ourselves.

All complementary medicines work by encouraging the body's inner healing resources. Whichever one we choose, we have to give it time to unfold and blossom. (That is not to say you should stick with anything which makes you unhappy. Tell your practitioner how you feel; ask questions and if you are not satisfied: change. There are many choices, and some things suit one person better than another. But before you choose the next thing, make sure you are willing to allow it to help you, rather than going along with the attitude: 'I don't believe you can help me, but you can prove me wrong if you like!')

I do know how depressing it is to doubt your practitioner and feel you would be well by now if only you had tried something else. When well-meaning friends question your choice and make other 'helpful' suggestions. When fears and doubts buzz around and around in your head. When you feel your practitioner simply hasn't done ENOUGH to help you.

Well, consider this: *Looking for the miracle pill is the way we try to hand over the responsibility of our illness to someone else.* Literally saying: 'I have all this pain and sickness, here it is, I want you to get rid of it for me'.

Just before Christmas, after I had been ill for four months, I became frantic and depressed to find myself still bedridden. I wanted to visit a friend: I wanted to be well enough to enjoy Christmas, and there I was: seemingly no better. I phoned my practitioner, begging her to give me another pill to cure me. I was convinced *there must be something*, she simply had not worked it out yet. She replied she had just given me a homeopathic remedy and I must give it time to work. Besides she was now on holiday, and as I was not an emergency she would not see me again until mid January.

I was hurt by her attitude at first, and resentful. But it was the best thing she could have done (as saying no—with love—is often the best thing) because it suddenly dawned on me: I was the only person who really cared whether I was ill or not, therefore I was the only person who could really help myself.

I began a routine of affirmations and visualisations (some are at the back of this book), I treated myself with acupressure.

But more importantly, I stopped looking helplessly outwards, towards others, for a cure.

Pill, treatments—even operations—are aids to help us get well. But it is up to you to make use of them. You are the one in pain, you are the one who needs to be well, and you are the one—and the only one—who can get yourself better. (Don't think I don't know what a cruel fact this is!)

Especially when we are weak and ill, in need of help and love, there wells up inside us a longing for a big hand to come out of the sky and put everything 'back to normal'. But help and love can only support us, it is not there to banish our suffering, to carry it off to some distant land. It is difficult to accept this, but when we were born on this earth, nobody promised us we wouldn't suffer.

There surely isn't a soul who can live through this life without experiencing suffering. Sometimes we have to suffer: *but*, (and this is a big but,) we can either make our suffering ten times worse by running away, being afraid, struggling against it, or we can look at our suffering and ask: "How can I learn from and grow through this experience?"

If we turn and open ourselves to our suffering, it may be that we discover hidden within that it is a gift, a deep and wonderful gift to our soul. A gift which—if we are truly able to appreciate—will enrich our life and bring us closer to our selves.

> Crisis or illness usually comes at a time of change, whether this is apparent to the person concerned or not. Indeed, one of the most healing things one can do is to draw attention to the fact that the origin of the word CRISIS (CHAOS) IS CHANGE and is therefore an opportunity rather than a disaster.
>
> (Christopher Greatorex)

If we chase after the Miracle Cure with such singlemindedness that we ignore the *process* of our illness, the question is: Is there something right under our noses that we are avoiding looking at? What is driving us on? *Why are* we so desperate? Do we want to go through life always feeling driven to be 'back to normal' and unable to face the pain and distress we know is

in our hearts? Don't we really long—in our deepest place—to stop for just a short while, to stop and to listen to our inner tears, and to comfort them, TO BE ABLE TO FACE OURSELVES.
To comfort ourselves.
To be comfortable within ourselves.
To heal ourselves from our sickness.

My eight year old son gave me one morning a bit of advice when I asked him desperately: "What can I do to get well?" He replied: "Perhaps if you enjoyed being ill, the bit of you that likes to spoil your fun would make you well again."

Sick in Bed

Oh these delicious hours
of peaceful surrender
time drifting by
a soft wisp of cloud

The pleasure of allowing
molecule upon molecule
to settle like dust
in the vast beat of the universe

To rest, and laze and turn
a somnolent *porpoise*
basking in the heat
of a warm comfortable bed

To come again to centre
all feelers turned inwards
a small ball of self
looking at Self

6

Performing Well

Look to this day, for it is life
The very life of life.
For yesterday is already a dream,
and tomorrow is only a vision.
But today well lived
makes every yesterday
a dream of happiness
and every tomorrow
a vision of hope.
                (From the Sanskrit)

Another day and you wake up again in bed, aching. Perhaps you have been waking on and off all night and in between dreams and glimpses of the darkness in the room, you have been aware of your pain.

Now you open your eyes, and slowly you grow conscious of something: you are still not recovered. It hits you with an awful sickness in the pit of the stomach. Perhaps you feel irritated and impatient. Perhaps you feel like crying. You try to think of something positive to cheer yourself up, but the thought is like a picture which keeps sliding out of focus. You swallow and try to grip on to the outside world: the colour of the sunlight on your bedside, the sound of rain.

You are afraid that inside is a terrible cry of panic which threatens to swamp you. You are afraid there is a dark stagnant well of despair inside and if you slip, if you let go of your precarious grip, you will fall down, down, and be gone forever. No one can help you now. Though people can be with you, people can help cure your body, people can even perhaps make you laugh.

You are ill and in your illness you are reduced to the centre of your being. And in the centre, along with all the beautiful parts of yourself, are all the other bits you don't want to recognise: the shadows, the selves you dislike, the unloved and hungry beings. This is not an easy place to be. And being ill, really allowing ourselves to stay in bed and be with ourselves in our discomfort, is not an easy thing to do.

Apart from the pressures we put on ourselves to be up and well, there is the fact that many of us have been used to putting up with 'not being 100%' for a long time, and we do not really know any more what real health (whatever that is for us) feels like. It is difficult to trust that by caring for ourselves just that bit longer, we can be just that bit better.

> In winter the life energy...is still underground. Movement is still at its beginning: therefore it must be strengthened by rest, so that it will not be dissipated by being used prematurely. This principle, of allowing energy that is renewing itself to be reinforced by rest, applies to all similar situations. The return of health after illness, the return of understanding after an estrangement: everything must be treated tenderly and with care at the beginning, so that the return may lead to a flowering.
>
> (The I Ching)

Every day the chances are that one of the questions you will be asked most often is: "How are you?" After you have been asked this for the ninth time you may find yourself feeling you should be able to report progress. "Much better thank you."

Gradually you may even begin to feel that you shouldn't just say you are better, but you should act as if you are better as well. This is a terribly hard thing. It simply is difficult to go on allowing ourselves as much 'tender treatment' as we need, and not to be drawn into 'performing wellness' to please (or even to prove something to) others.

We may temporarily make ourselves feel better too—it's nice to bask in people's smiles and appreciation when we appear to be 'up and about' again. But we may be asking for trouble. Performing well is wishful thinking. We know, really, when we do it, because we feel wobbly and delicate inside. Our getting up comes from our desire, our will power, and has nothing to do with a strong feeling of health urging our body to get up and out of bed. Once again we are caught up in the outer rings of our circle—caught up in the image we present to other people, rather than listening to ourselves.

In getting up and performing well we are following the part of us which says: "I can't stand it anymore, I am going to act as if the situation is different." And what are we avoiding? The part of us which says: "Help, I'm in need, I need to be acknowledged, I need to be loved, please help."

As clever and complex beings we can create very good reasons for anything we decide to do, very convincing arguments for any course of action. I have lain in bed many times justifying why I should 'perform well'.

Perhaps my muscles are deteriorating and I need to get up and exercise them!

Perhaps I can fight my way through the pain. If I just do what I want to do perhaps it will go away!

Perhaps I'm only so tired because I sleep so much!

Perhaps I'm not really in bad pain compared to other people, it's just that I'm weak-willed, and a hypochondriac!

Of course sometimes I have got up and tested these hypotheses, and nearly always been forced to admit that the pain is real, and I am genuinely weak and tired.

It is hard to be patient, but the most important thing to keep in mind is that, unless you die, you will get well again. In the moment when you feel yourself struggle with your pain, when you argue with yourself, when you feel the anxiety and guilt begin to gnaw at you: STOP, breathe deeply and say as you breathe in: "I" and as you breath out: "trust"

"I trust"

"I trust"

"I trust".

It is enough to know that through the shadows that lurk inside you, past the terrible voices, the forgotten parts of yourself, past the longing and the pain, is the core of yourselves, and that core is connected, as a baby with its umbilical cord to its mother, to the Divine Love of the Universe.

It is safe to be who you are, exactly as you are. You are created as part of the myriad pattern of life, and the pulse within your being beats with the same pulse as the pulse of life. "I trust".

A daffodil does not have to *do* anything to *be* beautiful. It grows in its tender beauty and blossoms glorious yellow whether it is in full view in your garden, or miles from human eyes, lost in a field full of other daffodils.

By being, it is being life. Just as you are.

7

Taking Responsibility

"My doctor told me to take 2 pills on an empty stomach."
"Did they do any good?"
"I don't know, they kept rolling off in the night."

Accepting that we are responsible for ourselves when we are ill—that no one can instantly cure us, that no one can feel our pain for us—is lonely but it is also invigorating.

When you come to the bottom line you find: it's none other than yourself. Yourself and how you relate to the world around you, the person within you, and the Divine (if you choose this at all).

One of the things which used to frighten me about dying was the knowledge that I alone would have to do it: I could be in a room full of loving friends and relatives, but only I would die. Only I would face the Huge Unknown. But when you come to think of it, the same is true of living: only I live my life. Only I look through my eyes. Only I feel with my senses. Only I have my pain.

Knowing I am my own 'bottom line' is not so awesome as it sounds because the vital thing is: it also gives me a lot of power to run my life, a lot of choice in how I run it, a lot of potential. You may not have chosen to be born the person you are, with all your faults and problems (though some people would argue that you *did* precisely choose) you may not want this present illness, but you can choose to use it.

Some of us are rather lazy, and unless life gave us jolts of some sort or another, we might tend to fall asleep, like Lewis Carroll's dormouse. But instead this pain or illness, which looked at first like being the worst thing that happened to you, turns out to be your friend, not your enemy.

Because it is your pain which has given you this opportunity to wake up, to take your dormouse head out of the teapot and look around the table, to notice who you're having tea with, to notice where you are sitting, and most of all to notice who you am, sitting here, and ask: how did I get here?

If I am responsible for myself, I have to be brave enough to look at my life and ask: is my illness trying to tell me something about myself? Is there something I need which I have not given myself? Is there an attitude towards myself or an approach towards life which I have that has led me to this bed?

Let me make this clear: this does not mean I am to blame for my illness. Blame does not come into it at all. I can't be to blame for my illness any more than I am to blame for being born who I am!

The tree grows on the side of the mountain, it grows short because of the strong wind; if the soil is poor, it grows thin and sparse, if the soil is rich, it grows bushy and strong. The tree is a tree. What use is blame to the tree?

There is no blame (no berating yourself, or criticising yourself—blame is a waste of time and attention. It is also a way of staying in feelings of guilt and self-pity rather than moving on to ask: OK, so if there is no blame, what do I do next?

The obvious place to start is with the part of you which has stopped you in your tracks right now. You were going along, feeling OK, at the very least managing, but your body knew better. Your body wanted something more from you, from life. And your body is you. You can't separate a tree from its trunk and leaves, nor can you separate a person from the body she inhabits.

The colour of your eyes, the shape of your limbs, the chemical make-up of your metabolism, all these factors go into shaping and making you the person you are. Your body is the vehicle with which you explore the planet. Your senses are the interpreters of life around you. Your limbs are the means you use to put your ideas into practice.

Further, the way you tense your muscles; the way you hold your head and limbs, the way you stand, the way you move: all these are expressions of yourself. A skilled therapist can tell an enormous amount about your life, not just who you are now, but about things that have happened to you in the past, simply by reading your body posture. Even your relationship to your parents, to love, to authority, to taking risks, all this is readable from the way you hold yourself.

This is *my* body. Yet how often do I remember to pay my body any attention? How aware are you of yourself right now? Wiggle your toes. Now wiggle your fingers. Squeeze your pelvic muscles. Wrinkle your nose.

Were you aware of those parts of yourself before? Do you feel that normally you live and move as if you filled all the frame of your body, right down to your little toes? Although we would find it hard to live on this planet without our bodies, many of us find actually being comfortable in our bodies is difficult. These little cartoons express some of the different attitudes I have noticed.

Some people ignore their bodies:

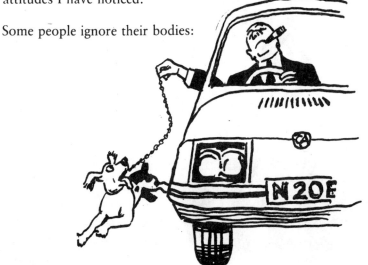

Some people bully their bodies:

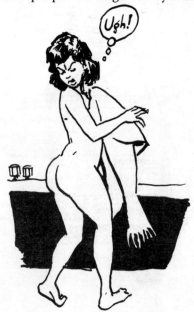

Some people are disgusted by their bodies:

Some people are afraid of their bodies:

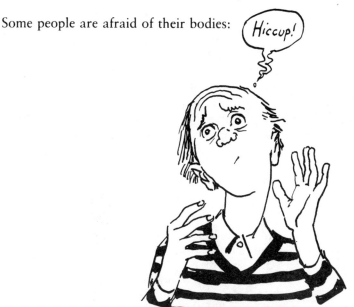

If we watch a young child, or an animal—a cat or dog, for example—we notice how easy they are in their bodies. Their joy in being themselves is the same thing as their joy in being in their bodies.

But somewhere during our growing up we begin to change. Perhaps we become engrossed in our education and we feel more identified with our minds than our bodies. Perhaps we are taught to feel ashamed of our bodily functions: perhaps we learn to hate the way we look; perhaps we have unpleasant experiences which make us afraid of our physicalness, and so gradually we think less and less about our bodies, care less and less for this part of ourselves.

> Our culture teaches us as we grow up that it's not alright to love ourselves. But there is a creative power that went to great trouble to put together the very delicate instruments we inhabit. What right has any of us to say: 'This old thing isn't much!' We should appreciate the beauty, the intricacy, the delicacy of the instruments that have been given us.
>
> (Paul Solomon: *Mind, Body, and Spirit*)

Be clear about this: the way we treat our bodies is the way we treat ourselves. If right now we are hurting somewhere in our body, and we ignore it, or become irritated by it—we are ignoring or being irritated by ourselves.

Illness is life's rather forceful way of making us see how vital our bodies are, how vital a part of ourselves they are. Hopefully, as a result we can begin to be more caring about the one and only vehicle we have to carry us through life.

My body is a sacred temple
through the corridors of bones
Thy spirit flows
In the beating of my heart
the pulse of stars and sea.
Each molecule, each particle
spirals a wondrous dance
around the altar of my being
dedicated to Thee.

8

Not Just Machines: Our Bodies

Consider a man washing his car on a Sunday afternoon. Picture him cleaning off the dirt, gently polishing in the shine. Especially if it is a nice day it will give him a great deal of pleasure to potter about fixing this bit here, polishing that bit there. He values the car, and he values his knowledge about it.

He knows, for example, how much air should be in the tyres, exactly which type of petrol it needs, which type of oil. He would not dream of trying to run a four star car on two star petrol. At the start of any long journey he will always check tyres, oil, water, battery fluid and so on.

Further, he listens out for the odd sound, that might indicate that all is not well. He knows for example, that running a car with a loose fanbelt puts extra pressure on the engine, and he would not dream of doing this for long. If a part wears out, he replaces it. If a part gets damp, he dries it. If a part becomes loose, he tightens it. He knows his car runs best under certain conditions, which, as he wants his to last, he tries to follow.

But how does the same man treat himself? Does he know —even—which conditions he needs in order to run at his best performance? Does he listen out for his parts going wrong so he can fix them *before* anything more serious happens? Does he spend a Sunday afternoon lovingly caring for himself?

Ask the average man that last question and you might be met by embarrassed laughter, although many men are fortunate enough to receive quite a bit of loving care from their wives or partners. But, do they know they need it? Do they give it to themselves?

And you, do you know you need it? Do you give it yourself? Do you even know *how* to give it to yourself, or *what* it is you need to be given? If you consider your relationship with your body, you may find that the only time you really notice it (except for making love, which in itself may be full of other complications as well as pleasure) is when you are in some way dissatisfied with yourself.

This may be either when you look in a mirror and decide you are too thin or too fat; or when you are ill and your body 'let's you down', and feels uncomfortable and unpleasant; or when you are tired, and you have to stop whatever you wanted to do on the insistence of sleep; or when your body is not good enough in some other way: will not lift enough, or move fast enough, or have an orgasm in the 'right' way... .

If we were bringing up a child, or even a dog, and the only time we noticed it was when we were critical of it, we would soon have a pretty mixed-up miserable dog (or child). Yet think for a moment over an average day during the time which led up to your illness. How much time did you spend actually enjoying the benefits of your body? By this I do NOT necessarily mean having sex, or indulging yourself in any special way—but simply remembering to enjoy such things as the *taste* of food, the *touch* of a child, or a tree, the *sound* of rain, or birdsong, the *feeling* of walking or dancing.

If you suddenly found your illness was terminal, you might find (as many people do) that you begin to appreciate all these simple joys for the gifts they are.

And now, lying in bed, there is no reason for you to ignore those of your senses which do work (your eyes, your ears, your taste, whatever). You could begin right now, in such a simple way to give yourself some enjoyment, some pleasure, right in the heart of your suffering.

Imagine you are a new born child. You have opened your eyes, and as no one has told you what anything is, your eyes are amazed by the vast array of colours around you. Try gently stroking your fingers over the bedcover, now feel the hardness of the table, or book next to you, touch your hair, explore the wonder of everything around you.

One of the reasons children enjoy themselves so readily is their ability to play with anything to hand—whether it is a stone, a cup, or a complicated toy. As we grow up we seem to lose almost completely the ability to enjoy what is to hand. We seem to spend most of our time chasing the things we are 'getting' or 'have to do'. While this desire to improve things and to create seems to be one of the instincts that makes humans what they are, as with anything else, something which is good can easily move to its opposite.

The more we rush after all the things—which we often call duties or responsibilities—the more we leave our body completely, and become totally engrossed in that outer layer of ourselves—the one connected to people and things outside ourselves.

This is one of the keys to our body: our body is our anchor to the present. Often along with old age and the slowing down of the body comes a greater ability to be in the present. But at any age we can learn to listen to the message of our body, and help ourselves keep our blood pressure down and our energy level up.

> Sometimes when I realise I'm really caught up in my thoughts or worries, I stop and remember to feel whatever it is I have in my hand, to notice whatever I'm walking upon, to smell the air, to breathe. This helps me come back to the moment. If I can catch myself at the point in the day when I feel all wound up and busy, with hundreds of things to do...and I take just a moment and stop, notice my breathing, notice my feet on the ground, unhunch my shoulders, I always feel calmer and more in control afterwards. When I get home at night I use this technique to leave the busyness behind. If I stop and simply listen with my ears, and feel the floor with my feet, and perhaps remember to smell a nice flower or something pretty soon I am really 'present' in my home, and able to enjoy whatever is right in front of me.
>
> (Catherine Savage)

It is with the body that I work as a teacher of the Alexander

Technique—a way of working with posture and movement to create a better balance and use of the body—and that last quote came from a client of mine. I am often filled with wonder at the beauty, intricacy, and outright common sense of our structures.

The design is so perfect: our bodies are built on the principles of balance and movement. The bones of the skeleton are like a building with each part balancing on the next. Then this is connected and kept together by our muscles, which curve round the frame of the skeleton in spirals. The muscle 'meat' is contained in a lining called fascia, and this lining goes all round the body. In this way every part of the body is connected to every other part.

The connection between every part of our body is also created by our nervous system: this is like a series of electrical fibres going down our spine, and then branching out into all the muscles like the roots of a plant. All the information received by the 'root ends' is fed back up the spine to the central computer: the brain.

There is no end of activity going on every minute. Not only are messages going back and forth, but our lungs are busy breathing and oxygen is busy being beaten into the flow of our blood by our pumping heart. The other organs of our body are also doing their jobs, so that secretions and other fluids are constantly squishing around. All this movement allows the intestines to massage our food down to our bowels. The picture is of a moving, changing body—perhaps not the still, boring object we imagine it to be. Of course the beauty is that we don't consciously have to monitor it to keep it going: we don't have to keep remembering to breathe, or beat our hearts, it all keeps going in the way as the sea keeps rolling in and out, in the same way new green shoots keep appearing out of the soil. The wonder of our living, moving body is like the wonder of our living, moving planet.

Providing we don't interfere, in fact, our body can function well. But most of us have habits of tension and posture which pull this fine structure out of shape. By hunching our shoulders and stiffening our jaw and neck anxiously, for example, we can

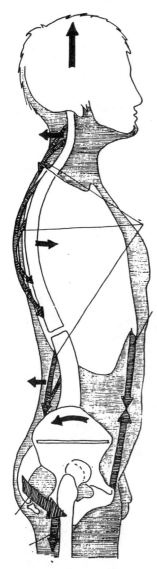
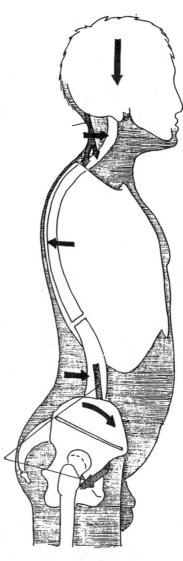

Lengthening of the Spine
(correct use of body)
the rib cage expands and
the abdomen less contracted

Downward Pressure
(poor use of body)
Notice pressure on lower back
and neck

collapse the whole of the body, creating pressures which gives us less air, less mobility. If we keep up these tension patterns year after year, the wear and tear on the body structure can have serious effects. If you think about the car, in the example at the beginning of the chapter, we would not dent and twist the car out of shape and expect it still to work properly. But we do expect out bodies to work, *whatever we do to them*, and we are often shocked if they don't.

One of the things I enjoy about my work is being able to explain to people that we do not just 'have a bad posture' 'have a stiff neck' 'have hunched shoulders'. We actually *do* them. Shoulders can't hunch (unless we are born without normal bones, muscles etc) unless we exert a lot of pressure on a lot of different muscles to keep them hunched. We may not know we

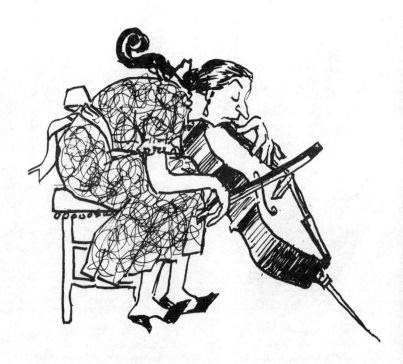

are doing it, in fact it probably feels quite normal to us, but the fact is that we put a lot of energy into keeping our muscles 'turned on' so the hunch can be maintained.

> The office worker, the conveyor belt engineer, the lorry driver, the mum-bent-over-the baby, the dentist, the pianist, carry out occupations for so long that they eventually will hold themselves partially contracted even when they are not involved in the actual pressures of their jobs. This residual tension may not be conscious, but eventually it is maintained most of the time. The summation of their various temporary attitudes eventually finds its expression in a posture—or a limited repertoire of postures, which come to dominate a person's character.
>
> (Wilfred Barlow: *The Alexander Principle*)

The important thing about all this is: realising that 'bad posture' is not something that hits us from outside, which makes us its victim. Instead it is something we learn and maintain through our own muscles, and can (no matter how old we are) unlearn.

The other point is: 'bad posture' is not really caused by things we do to ourselves, but the fact that we tend to pay more attention to our outer activities, to getting things done, than to our state of being, *the way* that we get things done.

For example: I go shopping. I am in a hurry and I concentrate on remembering and finding the things I need. I race around the supermarket with my mind on supper tomorrow night, the kids' dinners, screws for the wonky handle (I'm pleased I remembered that one), breakfast for next week... I pay at the cash desk with one eye on the time, and then suddenly I realise I have to CARRY everything I have bought.

I have been efficient and quick, my mind has raced from past to future, but the one thing I have overlooked is the here-and-now-problem of my strength (or lack of it) to carry out all my ideas. It is strange how so often looking after our body's basic needs comes way down our list of priorities.

When I was ill in bed my mother told me a story about a well-known Spanish Flamenco guitarist, who used to give

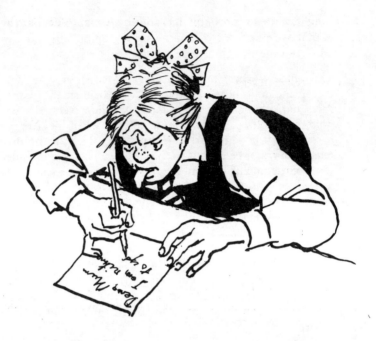

concerts all over Europe and every year he came to England.
Whether his concerts were organised by a large University or a
small guitar club, the story was often the same. He would turn
up beforehand, arriving (for example) at the lavish hall where
great care had been taken over the seating, the lighting, the
acoustics and, of course, on working out the finances. He
would discover that his simple requests—for heating so that his
hands did not get cold and he could play properly, for
something hot to drink,—had been totally overlooked.
"What?", he would ask in his expressive Spanish way "Who do
you think is giving this concert? Without me, there is no
music!"

For me this phrase is very to the point: "Without me there is
no music!" All the external things—as clever and attractive as
they might be—are only *trappings* to enhance the musician
him self. The first priority is to keep the musician fed and
warm so that he can play at all!

QUIZ: How do you rate as an ill person?

1. Your bedroom is your home for the next few weeks, do you:
   a) Lie there worrying about the dust, and who'll wash your next nightdress?
   b) Have all your favourite pictures brought in and decorate your walls with poems and inspiring sayings?
   c) Fill the room with plants, flowers, lovely music and beautiful smells?
   d) Draw the curtains and huddle up in your smelly sheets?

2. When visitors call, do you:
   a) Feel terrible that they can see you in such a state, apologise for everything, and wait for them to go?
   b) Get them to entertain you: telling you funny stories or having interesting discussions?
   c) Make yourself as attractively pale and wan as possible to encourage their love and sympathy?
   d) Not have or want visitors?

3. Lying there all day, do you:
   a) Find worries drift in and out of your head, each one more terrible than the last?
   b) Read as many interesting books as possible, watch TV and listen to the radio, and in the odd moment, write long extracts in your diary?
   c) Sew a beautiful tapestry while listening to Mozart?
   d) Stare at the wall?

4. The high spot of your day is:
   a) When the children/your partner comes in and helps you to smile and relax?
   b) Listening to 'Medicine Now' on Radio Four?
   c) Luxuriating in a wonderful scented bath by candlelight?
   d) Eating chocolates/guzzling beer?

5. To help yourself get well you:
   a) Take as many pills and remedies as you can?
   b) Devise a programme including diet, positive thinking and the appropriate treatment?
   c) Tell yourself as often as you can how lovely you are, laugh a lot, and use visualisations, prayer and/or meditation to create a good inner space?
   d) Eat chocolate, drink beer and smoke cigarettes?

6. When you are feeling low do you:
   a) Worry that you are not coping?
   b) Work out why: see if it is a habitual attitude dating from an incident in the past, work it through and try to cheer yourself up again?
   c) Wrap yourself in blankets, curl up round a hotwater bottle, and weep?
   d) Stare at the wall, eat chocolates, drink beer and smoke cigarettes?

There is no score, as all of us are only human.

9

Different Plants, Different Needs

Doctor: Your system needs toning up. What you should do is
take a nice cold bath every morning.
Patient: I do doctor.
Doctor: You do?
Patient: Yes, every morning I take a nice cold bath and I fill it
with nice warm water.

Not all illness is caused by neglect of our bodies, but if you are
honest you can probably find some aspect of your life that has
been neglected recently, which at the very least puts strain on
your health. We are complex creatures, and often it seems that
we can only satisfy one need at the expense of another: we get
the mental stimulation we need, and ignore our need for rest.
Satisfying our fear of the dark means we don't go out and then
we feel lonely.

More often it is a case of being caught up in providing the
basic requirements for living: our work, our home, our
children, other people's needs which lead us to feel we simply
can't 'afford' to give ourselves attention. Worst of all, some of
the ways we neglect ourselves are so habitual, so normal to us,
that we don't even notice we are doing it. Here are a few
examples of the way we can neglect our bodies, perhaps you
can recognise something of yourself!

Neglecting yourself because you are tired already.

The driver of this body feels there is not enough time, that there is too much to do, and she is the only one who will get it done. If she let go of the reins for a minute, everything would come tumbling down.

The driver is irritated because *other people should help*, but when they don't (or can't, because what they do is not good enough for her). Her response is to work harder as a punishment (but the only person she really punishes is herself). When she gets home at night, she is too tired to give herself the attention she needs. (If she can, she might blame someone else for not giving it to her.)

She promises herself rest in the future, but the future never comes; something always crops up. The body cannot continue this way forever, however, so it begins to complain gently at first, with a polite ache or pain. When this is ignored, the body—like any individual desperate to be noticed—shouts louder: It hurts, produces short term sharp pain which forces the person to stop in their tracks (e.g. migraine).

If ignored, it shouts louder still: with long term symptoms which should force the driver to slow down and take care. If this is ignored, the body, having done its best to warn her, keels over.

Neglecting yourself through sadness

The driver of this body is full of sadness. Sadness sits on her shoulder like a damp mist, and she keeps going, day after day, trying to avoid looking at it, hoping she can avoid being swamped. She cannot stop and listen to her body because she knows it stores all her pain, and she is afraid she will be swamped. She hides in her work, she hides in other people, in television.

But all the running away saps her strength, saps her desire for life. Feeding herself is difficult, nurturing herself in any way is hard because it gets too close. Either sleep is a welcome relief, or if she is unlucky, not even sleep is easy. One day this is bound to break. She can't go on running forever.

Neglecting yourself by taking a gamble

Though this driver's body has complained quite a bit lately, he doesn't take it seriously. In the past his body has always done him well. He has learned he can push his body hard, knock it about a bit (with alcohol, late nights etc), take a few risks and it pulls through OK

He is used to his body being strong and he won't accept there is any change. He feels it would be a waste of time listening to his body's complaints or going to the doctor. He laughs about it but really he wouldn't know how to cope if anything did go wrong. So he closes his eyes, and takes another gamble.

Neglecting yourself by not saying No

The most important thing to this driver is that he is liked. If there is no criticism he can feel safe. To be liked he has learned to think about other people to do things for them. So he does not pay much attention to any of his needs. But sometimes his body feels very tired, very dull and empty.

He doesn't try to find out why because he dreads the answer. The worst thing would be to have to say no. And yet the one thing he longs to do deep inside is to say no, and still be liked. He longs to be able to stop feeling everyone else is demanding something from him. He longs for a clear day. His body will express this longing. He will say NO by being ill.

All these people have reached a point in their lives where although something inside them needs looking at, they are so involved in their work, or family or other responsibilities, they cannot consider slowing down.

So they become more and more bound up in the needs of outer things (for example, the house, which needs repairing) and less and less aware of their own physical needs. They go on doing everything, assuming that their bodies can just keep up the pace.

But, you may rightly say, many of us find ourselves in jobs or circumstances where we can't do what we would like to do, can't meet our needs even if we knew what they were. Jobs, for example, where the machine (the check-out till, the automation line) is the priority, not the people running them. Homes too small for the number of children, flats without money to provide heat or comfort.

Yes. Of course this is true. As we are part of a society composed of people who have not paid their needs sufficient attention, we are under pressure to go along with the general habit. Given this situation we need have *some* choice, which is most often in how we approach the situation.

Mr. C says he will give me a job. As part of the job I have to hit myself on the head ten times a day. If I need the money, or if something else about the job interests me, I may choose to take it. While I am accepting his wages, I go along with this self abuse. (Of course I may try in various ways to point out to him that this distresses me, but that's another story.)

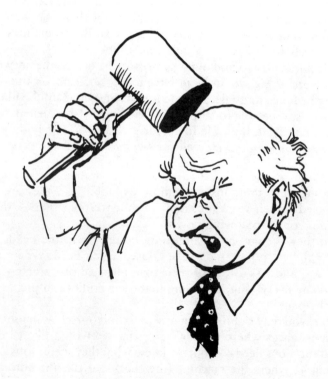

Now, what I have done is agreed to play his game in order to receive his money. But what I do not need to do—in any way—is to hit myself on the head when I am not at work. Or start to believe self abuse is right. Or start to believe that it is all I deserve. Or to believe that since I have been hit on the head, this gives me the right to do the same to other people. If I continue to know that I am worthy of praise rather than being abused, then those hits on my head can never harm my inner self, my spirit—though I may in the end decide the benefits of the job are not worth the headaches!

Obviously many times we put our work or other people first, not simply·in order to make money, or survive, but because we feel certain things must be done, certain needs have to be met. And we act in a way we believe is the best.

Surely there are times when you have asked yourself: do I need to do all this to be a good mother? Do all these jobs at work really have to be done this way? Very often if you look at these doubts you will discover you are trying to keep up to some ideal, some social value which you feel is 'The way things are done', a rule which may or may not be true, but is probably something you learned quite young and never inquired whether it suited your particular nature or not.

Like plants, we are all different; we have different needs for light and air, soil and water; different needs for rest and stimulation, company and isolation. In order for a plant to blossom, it has to have its needs met. The same is true for you. And your particular pattern is what makes you unique: it is to be respected, and loved, not squashed into some general rule, or hidden in shame or guilt.

Almost certainly you will have noticed that some of your needs are different from those of your friends, family or partner. Perhaps you wake up a grumpy bear while your partner is a chirruping lark. Perhaps you chill easily in cold weather. Perhaps you have a sensitive neck, or knee or elbow.

The beauty of life is that by getting to know ourselves well, we can give ourselves more and more of the things which make us feel good. What is the point in feeding yourself chicken if you would rather eat a mango?

Cycles

The Universe works in cycles: the water cycle of rain—streams
—rivers—seas—rising air—clouds—rain, being one. Dawn—
morning—afternoon—evening—night—dawn, is another. We
will have our own personal reactions to these cycles. For
example, some people find they get headaches just before a
storm, when the pressure is low.

For women, the idea of a cycle is easier to accept because
they know one particular cycle well: bleeding, awakening,
fertility, pre-menstrual, bleeding. But cycles apply to men as
well as women. The development of biorhythms was an
attempt scientifically to correlate some of these cycles, and
some countries take them far more seriously than we do here.
A simpler understanding of your most basic cycles is one you
can write down on a piece of paper right now.

First of all, consider the seasons: spring, summer, autumn,
winter. Most people have one season (mine is autumn) which
they really can't get along with: their energy feels at a low ebb;
they find themselves dreading its coming; it feels difficult for
them to carry on in quite the 'normal' way. There will also be
another season in which you find your energy level is usually
high. You find yourself looking forward to this season. The
other two seasons can be divided into a high-middle energy
season and a low-middle energy season.

Just take a moment and divide the seasons up as you find
them (You may assume everyone else finds the year the same as
you do, but if you ask, you might just be surprised). This is the
first cycle we respond to. Part of the year is a high-energy
outward-going time for us, part of the year is a low-energy
inward-looking time for us, and other parts balance in
between.

We can make use of this knowledge by, for example,
planning to start any outward, high energy project in our high
energy season, and using our low energy time to rest and
replenish ourselves, or to start a project which is more inward
looking and creative.

Next consider the monthly cycle. For a woman, or a man

who gets paid a monthly salary, this will be easier to notice. It may be if this idea interests you, you will actually take note over the next few months to find out how your cycle works.

Divide the month into four: (as before) low, low-middle, high-middle and high energy times. For many women the low energy withdrawing-into-themselves time coincides with the pre-menstrual week, but not by any means for all. This means that at some times during the month we may be more able to achieve certain things than at others. Rather than see ourselves as static personalities, we come to see that we change both our needs and our abilities from time to time.

Next consider the day. Each twenty-four hour period has two full cycles, and as such can be considered as two complete days. You will have your own individual low and high times, but most people find they fall into the general pattern.

Usually, sometime between awakening in the morning and early afternoon, each of us will experience a minor low; this is an interval for rest and nourishment. Then sometime between 3 and 7pm most of us will experience a major low. This may last longer (between 1–2 hours) and be more severe than the minor low, so it is imperative to nap and eat. We then experience another minor low sometime during the evening and another major low later on which is what

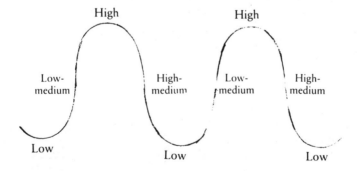

prompts us to go to sleep for the night. In between each of these lows is a low-medium, high and high-medium energy time.
(Swiftdeer, Deer Tribe Metis-Medicine Society)

Realising this pattern to the day is useful because it means we have something to plan around. It is no coincidence, for example, that many places of work have a small break at 11 and again at 3. You can also see that during your low hour of the day, in your low week in your low season you had better be extra nice to yourself and take extra care! You will not be so surprised if you feel depressed at this time, or completely exhausted and lifeless. Whenever possible you will plan nice treats: hot baths, massages, and plenty of rest.

The Natural Low Energy Times.
These are dream times, nagual times and times to pull in from activity and go into the 'creative-receptive' or 'feminine' mode. During our lows it is important to nurture and nourish the physical body through food, drink, relaxation, meditation and sleep...We must always honour our natural lows. If we overextend or push our energy during the low times, then our medium and high cycle energies will drop and our next low will be even lower. The low energy is like the energy of the West, the place of earth, introspection, magic, dreaming and death-giving life.
(Swiftdeer, Deer Tribe Metis-Medicine Society.)

Swiftdeer talks of 'honouring' our low times. Women often feel that their PMT, or natural low before their period is a nuisance, and a burden, and they struggle against it. What a different understanding it would be to *honour* this time of drawing-into-ourselves. Of nurturance and self-love, just as winter is the time of nurture for the earth and plants—so that life can come again from death—so that energy can come again from withdrawal.

Many of us have lost this idea of balance between low and high, life and death, withdrawal and going-outward. We want to emphasise the high and ignore the other. Yet it is an essential rhythm to life, and to us as living creatures.

Perhaps we are afraid of the low times because we have been taught to be afraid of failure, and these times feel too much like weakness, despair, depression. But of course if we nurture ourselves at these times, instead of criticising ourselves, they become times full of joy and good feelings. Any writer knows that good copy comes out of times of mental agony and depression. Any gardener knows that good plants come out of deep wet soil.

If we understand and trust cycles we know that darkness is the beginning of dawn, that nothing can keep going outwards, without going inwards. We can no more get stuck in the despair or confusion than we can in the outward positive joy. It is inevitable that the circle will turn, that the cycle will continue, that life will come of death, death of life.

> Your sorrow is your joy unmasked.
> And the self same well from which you laughter rises
> Was oft times filled with your tears.
> And how else can it be?
> The deeper that sorrow carves into your being
> The more joy you can contain.
>
> (Kahlil Gibran)

It is through the fermenting, through the long days nurtured in the dark womb, that whatever is waiting to burst forth from us, forms itself, and becomes ready to blossom.

10

Understanding Energy

One of the things I found helped me most to get well was understanding energy. Or, to put it another way: one of the reasons I went on being ill for so long was because I didn't understand energy.

When I was twenty-one I had an operation, and afterwards I found myself in debilitating pain. Being young and extremely strong willed I found it VERY difficult to allow myself the conditions I needed to cure myself. Basically, as soon as I felt the slightest bit well I went out and did as much as possible, until at some point I inevitably did too much, when the pain would become so ferocious that I would be stopped in my tracks, and have to rest up again.

When I rested I would be morose and sorry for myself; I would look at all the people in the world and think: why do I have to be ill and crippled when I could get so much out of life? Why didn't it happen to Mary who doesn't want to go mountaineering anyway? Or Sarah who doesn't like dancing all night long?

The resentment would build and bubble, so that by the time my body was even one quarter well, I would be like a bottle full of gas, and off, off I would go: desperate to do all the things my illness had prevented me from doing, and the cycle would start again. It sounds funny, but it was a serious stage of affairs because I was ill and in pain, nearly constantly, for nine years, and through my behaviour my system became seriously debilitated.

A Chinese acupuncturist, whom I went to after a few years of this, tried to explain the rudimentary principles to me. "Tessa", she would say, "What you do is to spend £10 when you only have £8 in your bank account." Unfortunately I never really understood her—I thought she was telling me I should rest more, or sleep more, or lead what I saw as a boring, unproductive life; spending all my time putting my body first and never having any fun.

The point I missed completely was that it was not a case of resting more, and then going at it full pelt again whenever I was active, but of being more aware of all the energy I frittered away during every hour I was awake.

Basically there was no *peace* in me. I had to be doing something. My mind had to be worrying about something, and my emotions had to be turned full on over some issue or other. And all at once, too. I was wound up, like a taut spring. My mind was overly busy and my muscles in a permanent state of tension. If I had any concept of my centre I couldn't stay with it, because being there seemed to face me with my weakness. I felt expressing my feelings was a release, but as they were so often anger or sadness and so rarely laughter and joy, expressing my feelings only added to my being in a bad state.

This may sound as if I was quite loony, but had you met me I would have appeared fairly normal, quite in control of myself (even fairly likeable). It is my experience that an awful lot of people (in the West anyway) go through life in a state at least nearly as bad as the one I was in.

Another side of my character was that I was very generous with my time and energy. I liked people, and spent a lot of time with them—often finding myself listening to their problems and trying to help solve them. This made me feel I was stronger than most other people, and I was happy to be able (as I saw it) to 'give', though I sometimes felt nobody understood what I was suffering.

Actually, although maybe I did offer some good advice, the real fact was I needed people, and I needed to feel stronger than them because I didn't want to face the small needy part in myself.

Another thing was that I was deeply moved by all the suffering in the world (I still am, but in those days the thought of suffering actually made me feel physically hurt, and worse, full of helpless outrage and anger, which seemed to bubble and boil inside me like poison), but the more I concentrated on it, the more helpless I felt in the face of its vastness, and the more angry I was.

I understood that being angry and upset by things which were beyond my control was *not good for me* on a daily basis, but I didn't believe I could change my state (or that it was morally right for me to change it) until the world had changed. My Chinese acupuncturist once said to me: "You cannot save a drowning man by jumping in beside him and drowning with him."

I was very struck by that phrase and it help me a good deal. But I still wanted to find out how I *could* save the drowning man, and the only way seemed to be by being strong: by being so clever and such a good swimmer that I could help everyone who came in touch with me. The intention was an honourable one, but to begin with I was not and am not a saint, and in fact am physically weaker than the average person, having been born with a small frame and scoliosis of the spine. Besides, my thinking—though coming from genuine love and care—was warped by my ego, and really showed a need to be thought wonderful, and to be needed by others.

When I began my training to be an Alexander Teacher I was lucky enough to meet a teacher who stopped me in my tracks. "What about the starving and tortured person in yourself?", she asked me. I feigned disbelief, but the words stuck and from that moment I began the journey into looking at what really is: into learning to love and care for myself, and through that discovering the universal or Divine Love which surrounds me. When I realised the Divine Love is very strong and very loving, I realised there was no need for me to try and be a poor substitute.

It seems to me when I look at people—in particular

women—that many of them are like containers which leak all over the place. They need others to give them love, but no sooner is it poured into them than it begins to leak out again.

Most of us feel uncomfortable about being *full up*. We are afraid of being greedy or selfish. We feel we should keep giving to justify ourselves. This is not real Christianity as Jesus taught it, because one of the things about him and his disciples was that they were strong, full people. We may feel that by giving we are doing our Christian duty, but it is only by being full in ourselves that we can really begin to be of use to the Divine. Otherwise we get stuck in the pattern of living constantly on borrowed energy, needing more and more so that we can pass it on again, so that people think we are good (or wonderful), so that we can avoid looking at the panic and neediness inside.

As long as we live out this pattern, we will go through life never feeling particularly well. Only if we can allow ourselves to be 'full' can our healing begin.

Take a moment now and imagine an egg. Increase the size of the egg in your imagination until it is an egg-shaped container two feet in height. Now imagine the container is in the body of a person, nestled onto the floor of the pelvis and on up until the top sits underneath the rib cage. Allow the person containing the egg to have a head, and arms and legs. Visualise that the container is nearly empty. There is dryness and heat. The person has a temperature. There is cracking around the edges of the egg. The person is in terrible pain. They are very ill.

Imagine the container fills up with a liquid like water mixed with light until they are one quarter full. Feel how soothing this liquid is. See how the light gives the person enough energy to open their eyes. To move their arms, and even to open their mouths and eat. This person still feels very delicate and ill, but they have enough energy to do the most basic things (eat, go to the toilet etc). They are still in pain. Visualise more water and light going into the container, until it is half full. Feel how there is now a substantial weight in the bottom of the egg: the person feels more 'solid'. The water is very clear and beautiful. The light is so golden that it shines almost up to the dark ceiling of the egg. The person is now well enough for basic survival. Their pain may diminish somewhat because the body will begin to use any spare energy to start to heal them.

It was at this point I always used to imagine I was well, and start to get up and about. Immediately the energy which was going into healing me had to be used to achieve all the other things I started to do, and pretty soon—leak, leak, leak—I was back to quarter full and back in bed. The important thing is that when you are half full with energy, you continue to act as you did when you were quarter full: just eat, rest and enjoy resting. Then the *maximum amount of energy* can go into repairing your illness.

Now imagine more water and light filling the egg until it is three quarters full. The vibrancy of the water and light now begins to show on the outside of the person's body so that he begins to look better. The light now reaches up to the roof of the egg, and can begin to repair all the dark places. Repair work is still going on everywhere, though the person may begin to feel much better.

At this point far too many people count themselves well. Pressures of work and finance, of children and a house needing care add to the inner pressure for the person to 'act well'. It is here that the balance is most precarious. The person can get up and about, but must be careful not to put the system into top gear. And yet, because he feels fairly well, he may slot into his old pattern of doing things and completely ignore his body again. Besides, not knowing what it feels like to be full, a person may not expect any more. And often he feels he now has enough to start giving it away, and so—leak, leak, leak—back he goes: half full, even a quarter full. Perhaps not even the original pain, but colds, flu, glandular or hormonal disturbances, which tell him (if he would only listen) that his system is still vulnerable.

Now imagine the container totally full. The clear water touches every wall, making it flexible but solid, healing each cracked surface. The light in the water now shines through the eggshell, and out from the person's skin. He appears 'glowing with health', 'vibrant', 'full of energy'. At this point there is enough energy for the final healing stages to continue, while the person also goes about his life.

The important thing is: no one can have a full egg unless he has learned about listening to his own needs, until he is able to say no, until he is able actively to choose which ways they spend his energy, until he is able to *contain*.

11

Limits

He who stands on tiptoe is not steady.
He who strides cannot maintain the pace.
He who makes a show is not enlightened.
He who is self-righteous is not respected.
He who boasts achieves nothing.
He who brags will not endure.
According to the followers of the Tao
"These are extra food and unnecessary luggage".
They do not bring happiness;
Therefore followers of the Tao avoid them.

Becoming ill is one way of being shown our limits. It is not a pleasant way, but sometimes the best lessons we learn are not ones we enjoy at the time. If we put our hand in the fire and discover it burns, we know not to do it again. With any luck we learn the limits of our skin and the nature of the world we inhabit without losing our hand.

It can be very demoralising to realise we are not as strong as we wanted to be. It feels very depressing to realise we have (at least temporarily) to let go of some of the things we wanted, because we are not strong enough to get them.

If we have been 'standing on tiptoe' we were bound to lose our balance in the end. If we were juggling more balls than we could handle, we were bound to drop one in the end. It is very hard to realise we are mortal, and that if we push ourselves

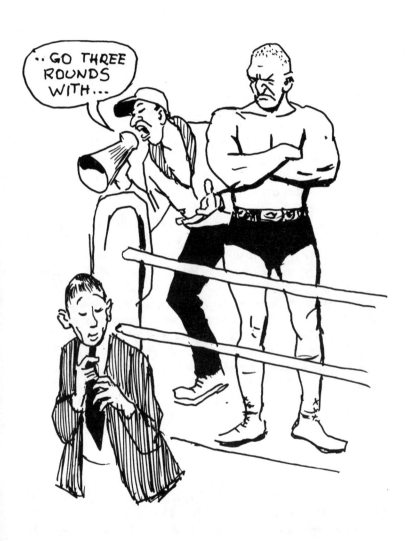

beyond our capacity, we will die. It is hard to realise that we are human, that we can't neglect any part of us for too long without something giving way. It is hard to accept our limits, but the saying goes: 'A wise man knows his limitations'.

Sometimes it is not just our own limitations we have ignored, but the limitations of life around us as well. Perhaps we were swimming upstream, in the strongest water flow rather than going more gently by way of the shallows and rock pools. Perhaps we were driving too fast, and left too many things behind. Perhaps we had not weighed up all we were taking on, and the last brick came as a surprise.

Containment is important because it means we stop spilling out all over the place and do not overstep ourselves. Part of being contained is trusting that it is as good to say NO in life as it is to say yes.

Saying NO is a way of choosing what life will bring to you. It is a way of daring to expect that something better is on the way; of trusting that if we don't go speeding down the first road we come to, we may be led to a far more interesting destination.

Accepting your limits is not the same as denying life. Often we deny life's opportunities because we're scared that someone else will damage us, by not respecting our limits. But if we know our limits, we can say NO and protect ourselves. If we know our limits we can feel safe when we say YES.

Saying NO is definitely a vital part of getting well. Perhaps you are hardly recovered, but someone offers to take you out of your boring old bedroom, out to a party. To cheer you up, they say. Although you would like to go, you say NO, you are not well enough.

Later on a friend calls round and you spend a lovely time together. Or a great programme comes on the TV. When you next meet the person who asked you to the party, the chances are they'll say: "Oh, you didn't miss much!"

It can feel difficult and 'weedy' to say NO to other people. It can feel hard to put ourselves and our health first. But just as we learned and grew when life gave us a big NO (when we became ill), so NO is just as much a helpful word to say to someone as YES. We may feel we can help person X by doing something for him, but perhaps it would be more help to him if he learned to do it for himself.

This is not a way of telling you not to help others, or not to care for or love others. But if the others care for you, they will not wish you to 'ruin your health' by helping them anyway. Often one person does things for another and it helps neither of them. Have you ever gone somewhere with a friend for his sake, only to find when you get there that he was doing it for *your sake*?

Provided you say NO to help yourself, and not in order to hurt the other, no harm will come of it. Giving comes when we can give freely with no thought of return. How can we give freely if our energy egg is only three quarters full—whatever we give away we are going to need back again from someone else! "Do unto others as you would have done unto yourself." To act in this way, you have to 'do unto yourself' first so you know what it feels like!

12

Worry Patrol

Patient: Doctor! Doctor I think I'm shrinking!
Doctor: You'll just have to be a little patient.

One of the distressing aspects of lying in bed is that the voice in your head which likes to worry is given eons of time to do so. Or at least, having a lot less to do, you find yourself having to listen to it. Sometimes the worry voice can almost drive you mad. With every worry it puts forward you feel your stomach churn, and your heart wrestles in your chest.

"Maybe I will never..."

"What if it...?"

"How will I manage...?"

"What if I don't...?"

Of course you would stop worrying if you could, but the voice is so persistent. It is impossible to defend against it at all times, and any unguarded moment: there it is again.

In a way worrying is perfectly natural; being in an unsettled state of mind is part of your illness. Feeling vulnerable and out of control is part of having no reserves. But there *are* plenty of things you can do about worrying. The first is to realise that although you may be worrying more than usual, that worry voice is not a stranger to you. Anything you are experiencing now is simply an increase of things you tend to do anyway —even if you usually ignore them.

The second thing you can do is exactly what you don't wish to do: listen to the worrying voice. But instead of letting the voice swamp you and make you sick, you are going to make a space so that you don't get too close. Begin this with your breath. Each time you feel too close to the worry voice, STOP, listen to your breath, breathe deeply, and breathe again. This should distance the voice again.

Now you are going to listen to your worrying voice as if it is a stranger. A stranger talking to you. Although we know the worry voice is you—at least part of you—in order to hear it the important thing is to avoid *identifying* with it. If you identify with the voice it will pretty soon swamp you, and you won't be able to listen any more. But ironically, if you stay at a distance from the voice, you will be able to listen to it, and be more objective and clear about what is being said. As the voice speaks to be heard, not to be evaded, it would actually prefer you to distance yourself if that is the only way it can get to speak to you.

Perhaps you can start by just listening for a minute at first, and then stop, look out of the window, or come back to the book. If you notice yourself feeling terrible when the worrier starts to speak: STOP. Breathe. You are getting too close. Distance yourself and start again.

The easiest worry-banishing exercise is the following one. It is really a kind of taking-the-bull-by-the-horns.

Begin by asking the worry voice to name one (the main) worry. For example: 'I'm worried about my work.' Ask the worry voice:

"Why are you worried about your work?" He'll reply, perhaps: "I'm worried John won't cope with everything."

Now the purpose of this exercise is to take the worry through *to its worst extreme*. So keep asking questions that *draw out* more of the worry.

"What will happen then?"

"If John doesn't cope with everything, I'll lose clients."

"And then?" (Keep breathing)

"If the business folds I won't be able to pay for our house."

"And then?"

"My wife and children and I will be turned out on the streets, we will be destitute."

"And then?"

"We will be a shame on the family name. We will be reduced to begging."

Now picture yourself begging. Picture your cupped hands. Picture the huge starving eyes of your wife and children...and with any luck you'll laugh. Yes, laugh. Because taken to that extreme it's ridiculous.

Next, while you are in a better humour, point out to your worrier all the other options; don't reign-in your imagination; let yourself say the wildest things.

"I could sell up and buy a yacht and sail to the West Indies with my wife and children."

Allow yourself to get into the fantasy and enjoy it. As you are stuck in bed for a while, be you own movie and really enjoy the West Indies. This approach can be applied whatever worry you have; For example:

"I'm worried my child will not be looked after properly."

"I'm worried someone will find out and she'll be taken into care."

"I'll be called a bad mother and I'll never get her back."

"I'll get so angry about it I'll get up out of bed and go to the office and attack everyone and then I'll be sent to prison where I'll get even more ill..."

Once you have worried yourself near death and in prison you can see the Shakespearean proportions your worries can take, see that life is unlikely to treat you this way, in this country, if you become unwell.

Now instead, try other options:

"I'll contact the social worker who'll turn out to be brilliant, and she will find her a place in that crêche I've been trying to get her in."

"My mother will come up and look after us both, and we will finally make up all the arguments we've had in the past, and be real friends at last."

Really indulge these thoughts too. Remember the things you

love about your mother. Remember the times people have turned out better than you'd feared.

I am not saying it is easy: if you are a single parent of a young child, and you find yourself ill and alone, my heart goes out to you. You are being tested to the limits of your endurance. But someone up there knows you can cope with it, knows that whatever experience you have, you will use it to grow and help others. Don't forget to ask for help: and trust that even in your situation you *can* help yourself. In fact in your situation you may *have* to help yourself, and stripped to the bones you will come up again, because this is your gift.

Once you have laughed at the worry, and played with other alternatives, you may find the obvious solution simply comes drifting into your head. Or you may find that your worry voice is quite put out at your solving the problem, and will immediately start again on a new one. Our minds are best at one main task: problem solving. In order to solve problems, your mind has to think up problems to be solved in the first place. Worrying is simply your mind taking it's job too seriously.

Having a full-blown worry and giving yourself the opportunity to enjoy it may satisfy your worry voice's need for self importance for a bit, and give you a moment's respite.

Peace and relaxation. When we are ill, the most healing moments for us are those when we can feel *at ease*, safe, satisfied. This is why many people find reading or knitting such a good occupation during illness: it take them into a safe and interesting world, away from difficulties and fears.

When we are ill we need to try to achieve some kind of balance between—plenty of times when we are feeling safe and at ease, and—times when we look at our fears and needs and worries and try to satisfy them (or least listen to them) so that we are not supressing problems which will only try to surface again sooner or later. Worrying is an unpleasant pastime. But it serves a purpose. What can worrying give us?

Help to get rid of fears
Sometimes no amount of logic can banish our deepest fears.

We know they are ridiculous, but we need to voice them. A friend who understands this and lets us pour out worry after worry until we have exhausted them, is worth her weight in gold. She does not identify us with our worries, or put us down for having them. She does not even try to solve them. She understands the therapeutic value of *naming the worst*. (As we did in our worry-banishing exercise.)

Worrying, in this way, is simply a bringing-fear-to-the-surface, and the sense of relief we feel afterwards is the reason we do it.

Worrying as a way of nurturing

It could be that during your childhood you learned that worrying is a way of showing love. When Mum said: "If you don't do up your coat you'll catch your death of cold!" her worrying meant that she cared about you: she didn't want you to get a cold or die, and so forth.

If you listen to the worry voice in your head you may recognise this quality in it: you worry as a way of *trying to care for yourself*. It may not be the most helpful way to care for yourself (as the phrase 'sick with worry' makes clear) but if you can see the GOOD INTENTIONS behind the worry voice, perhaps this will help you feel better about this part of yourself.

Next time you worry, see if you can find out what care you are really trying to give to yourself.

Worrying as a way of going for the best

Another motive behind your worrying may be this: you are worrying because you care that everything should go alright; that you do your best to make things turn out right. You are so very keen to do your best, but the way you measure your success is by criticising yourself: worrying about everything you have done wrong, or everything which might go wrong in the future. In other words what started out as a fine motive: going for the best, has become a stick to beat yourself with. No one performs at their best while they are being beaten with a stick, let alone gets much enjoyment out of life.

The finer and clearer the *ideal* we have about how life *could be*, the more ammunition this gives the part of us which wants to criticise and improve ourselves. The trouble is, just as the nature of an ideal is that it is beyond our daily reality—so the nature of our personalities as human beings is that WE ARE NOT PERFECT. We all need time to just let ourselves ENJOY BEING WHO WE ARE, FAULTS AND ALL. Of course it is one thing to know this, and another to explain this to the bossy and very critical voice in our heads!

Gestalt therapy deals with the problem of our critical voices by *separating them from ourselves*. (Just as earlier we listened to our worry voice by distancing ourselves from it). A Gestalt therapist will literally separate the voice by suggesting the person sit on one chair (or cushion) and identify and act out one voice, and then move to another chair, and act out and identify with another voice. The important thing is that the voices TALK TO EACH OTHER.

For example if we were with such a therapist, and were looking at our criticiser voice, we would sit on one chair and identify with the voice, giving it permission to speak. We would look at the other cushion—as if we were addressing ourselves—and say (for example):

"You're not good enough..."

"You did that wrong...'

and so forth. Then we would swap over to the other chair and try to communicate with the voice:

"It hurts me that I'm never good enough for you..." (Or whatever we wanted to say.)

To explore this thoroughly, of course, you need to have the help of a Gestalt therapist. But the understanding which might be of some use to you now is this: the voice is only one part of you. You have another part of you who can answer the voice back, or laugh at the voice, or tell it when its being too hurtful. Just being aware that the criticiser *is not always right*, and that anyway IT IS ALRIGHT TO MAKE MISTAKES (which often turn out for the best), may help too.

Perhaps you could take a moment and write down some of the standards of behaviour you think you should keep to. Ask yourself, would I expect this of anyone else? Would I expect this of someone sick in bed?

Worrying as a way of avoiding 'now'

Sometimes worrying, going over and over this and that, may seem to be a less painful option to our unconscious mind, than accepting the *truth*.

If, for example, we spend time worrying about our work, we are avoiding accepting the fact that we are not at work, and *can't be at work*. We are still clinging onto the idea of work, and our identification with it, rather than letting it go and looking at ourselves here and now.

Sometimes asking ourselves when we find ourselves worrying: 'What is this worrying helping me to avoid?' may help put things in perspective. For no matter how uncomfortable it may seem, facing the truth brings with it such relief afterwards. A truly wonderful healer I know taught me: 'TRUTH IS THE ONLY HEALER.'

The moment we face a truth we feel good, at ease, expansive, comfortable, at peace. These are the states of being that are most likely to heal us. Running away from truth takes so much energy: fear, tension, screwing ourselves up, convincing ourselves, denying things, and so forth. Khrishnamurti puts it this way:

> There is no such thing as a problem, only a truth we cannot face.

13

Ideals

Patient: Doctor, Doctor!. I keep thinking I'm a curtain.
Doctor: Pull yourself together.

Ask your mind to build a bridge from here to the moon and it
has done it in the time it takes you to imagine it. What's more it
can equally quickly imagine what the bridge is made of, who is
allowed to go on the bridge, what reward there will be for
building it, and so on.

There is not limit to to the visions our minds can have. This
is a wonderful aspect of the mind—from this come stories and
plays, paintings and new inventions. All the same, just because
we can imagine something does not make it practicable.

Ideals are another kind of vision we have, something beyond
daily reality. An ideal is as it says: not real, but larger than real.
By it's very nature it is something we can work towards but not
obtain. Long before we got to the actual place of our ideal, our
mind would be able to imagine another ideal, way beyond.

The nature of this aspect of the mind is that *it goes beyond*.
Because it goes beyond it interests and excites us. But we often
seem to forget we can never live up to our ideals, we çan never
create in a material way everything we can imagine. Sometimes
we make ourselves ill chasing a vision. Sometimes we destroy
ourselves (or someone else) comparing ourselves (or them) to
an ideal. Although the visions and ideals glitter like hidden

gold, tantalising to our prospecter selves, they also serve a negative purpose: they keep us from seeing, living and enjoying what *really is*.

You may not notice that half the things you believe in are, in fact, ideals. Take your code of moral behaviour. Is this an ideal, or something you can act out daily? Take your picture of your perfect partner (or the way you'd like your existing partner to behave)—is this an ideal, or could he or she really be like that?

It does not matter how exactly your ideals have captured what you believe in, how good or clever they are, if you don't see them for what they are: ideals. And ideals, by their very nature *can't* exist in reality. If they did we might discover they were not as perfect in practice as they seemed in our heads!

The following story is one that has been told in many forms by many different storytellers:

> Once upon a time there was a man who was an inventor, and he decided to create his ideal woman. He invested all his life's savings in the materials he needed, and shut himself away in his laboratory. Day after day he worked obsessively on his task. He did not notice the food he ate, nor the clothes he put on, so absorbed was he in his work.
>
> Outside his stuffy laboratory the birds sang. The summer sun ripened the corn which danced a merry dance against the bright azure sky. The man continued to work obsessively. He worked late into the night, and found he had trouble sleeping. He became agitated and morose. He longed to complete his task, but things would keep going wrong, forcing him to work long and hard to calculate solutions to his problems.
>
> Autumn with its golden leaves and melancholy sunshine turned into the softly drizzling days of early winter. Snow came, crisp still whiteness covering the earth. The man was cold in his laboratory, because he spent his money on materials not on heat. But he didn't mind anymore, didn't mind that he had next to nothing to eat, and his clothes unwashed. He was in a state of feverish excitement: his experiment was nearly finished.

One dark winter's morning the invention he had made came to life. Ah, she was beautiful. Ah, she was a joy to behold! The inventor sat back in his chair and watched her with great satisfaction as she walked obediently around the room.

But as the hours passed he began to notice all the ways she did not exactly match his ideal. Gradually her faults seemed more and more obvious to him. What should have been a time of great celebration for him, began to dissolve into bitter dissatisfaction. Soon he had turned his machine off, and had started once again with improvements.

I don't need to continue the story because I'm sure you understand the gist of it. While the beauty of real life is all around him, our inventor fixes on an ideal which will never satisfy him. He denies his health, his sanity, his ability to enjoy pleasures because he feels the thing he is chasing is the most important thing.

But we know, of course, that it will go on evading him forever, for he is misusing the ability of his mind to create ideals, and to bring a part of these ideals into reality. The important fact he has not appreciated is: *the way in which he goes about his tasks is part of the task itself.*

When you are lying in bed you may find your mind likes to torture you with ideals and ideas about *any aspect of your life you are presently unable to participate in.* If you can't work, your mind will tantalise you with pictures of all the amazing achievements which would have happened had you worked, with all the opportunities you have missed and so on. The same will be true about college, or bringing up children.

The point to realise is: these are ideas, not true pictures. Very rarely (if ever) does life work out as we imagined it would. We simply can't take into account all the hundreds of variables. But if we believed our minds, we could have a field day concentrating on our worries, most of which are not accurate anyway.

An example of this comes from my last illness. As the sole person responsible for my child I had to be (most of the time) father and provider, mother and friend. Suddenly, being ill, I was able to be none of these things. Luckily in the early stages, grandparents from both sides came to my rescue. Far from being a disappointment for my child, this was a real treat for him.

During my long convalescence I was often tired, and I feared that he suffered because I couldn't fulfil all the ideas I had for him: playing games together, earning money to buy him nice clothes or toys, being able to take him out at weekends. But in fact the illness changed our relationship for the better in a way *I could never have imagined*. For my son—who has always had a working mum—having one constantly at home was wonderful. I learnt to listen to him better—because I had less energy to talk. He spent a lot of time reading to me—because I couldn't read to him, and his reading improved in leaps and bounds.

If I had believed all the worries my mind could dig up, I might never have appreciated the reality staring me in the face: that everything was more than OK, it was all happening for the best.

> There is for each man, perfect self-expression. There is a place which he has to fill and no one else can fill, something which he is to do, which no one else can do; it is his destiny!
>
> This achievement is held, a perfect idea in Divine Mind, awaiting man's recognition. As the imaging faculty is the creative faculty, it is necessary for the man to see the idea, before it can manifest.
>
> (Florence Scovel-Shinn: *The game of life and how to play it*)

To recognise that our mind can sometimes fool us, and that our ideas can, instead of enlightening us, actually make us feel frustrated and critical, is *not* to reject the value of the imaging part of our mind, or the value of having an ideal to aim for.

We have an incredible and powerful tool in our heads! Most of us haven't even begun to explore it's full potential. A trick I learned when I was young was that instead of using an alarm clock, if I needed to wake at a certain time in the morning all I had to do was bump my head against the pillow as many times as the hour I wanted to wake at (seven times for seven o'clock) and sure enough at seven I would wake!

I recently taught this to my son, and it worked for him too. I have also taught him to transfer any of his small aches and pains into a crystal, and so be healed. This also works for him, because he believes it will, and as I have never told him anything else, and as he has experienced it for himself, it will continue to work, and as long as he goes on believing it (or, one could say, trusting in the healing power of a crystal).

In the same way if we go on imagining that our fears and worries are true, we can imagine them into existence.

> Keep thy heart (or imagination) with all diligence, for out of it are the issues of life. (Proverbs 4:23)
>
> This means that what man images, sooner or later externalizes in his affairs. I know of a man who feared a certain disease. It was a very rare disease and difficult to get, but he pictured it continually and read about it until it manifested in his body, and he died, the victim of distorted imagination.
>
> (Florence Scovel-Shinn)

The mind is a very powerful tool, thought a vital part of life. Some people go as far as to say that life is only as it appears to us, because we imagine it that way, and if we changed our thoughts, life would change accordingly. Shamen talk of 'dreaming the dream', keeping the world in the shape we wish to keep it with the power of our mind.

Whatever we believe, it is certain that our mind can be used far more than most of us tend to. This is where the idea of positive thinking comes in: the notion of changing our thoughts consciously (changing our mind with our mind) from a negative picture to a positive picture.

Consider for a moment: how often during the day do you have thoughts flitting through your head, almost too quick to notice, such as: 'I'll never get well now', 'The pain is getting worse', 'This headache is too much to bear'. There's nothing wrong with thinking these thoughts provided that when you think them, you notice them. If they are serious (such as my headache is too much to bear) they deserve immediate attention. With a cry for help, you need comfort and nurturing.

Treat yourself in the way I describe in Chapter sixteen, 'Listening to our other parts'.

However it may be you are simply in the habit of saying things to yourself without noticing you do. And so, without being aware of it, you are feeding negative thoughts all day long into your computer. 'I am in pain. I won't get well' and so on.

Now our computer is an obedient tool and it will do its best to keep to your word. Your negative thoughts are important: they are having an effect on your health!

But if our negative thoughts can effect our health, so can our positive ones. When we are ill it is difficult, if not impossible if the pain is especially bad, to stop the fear and worry and simply be positive. In fact trying to do this would just be phoney. But what we can do is notice the next time we say: "Oh this pain, it hurts so", and quite consciously add: "But it is getting better."

In other words we cancel the power of the negative thought, and put in a positive direction instead. Just doing this feels quite good immediately, but it is more powerful than that.

> The imagination has been called 'The scissors of the mind' and it is forever cutting, cutting, day by day, the pictures man sees there, and sooner or later he meets his own creations in his outer world. To train the imagination successfully, man must understand the workings of the mind...
>
> There are three departments of the mind, the sub-conscious, conscious and superconscious. The subconscious is simply power, without direction. It is like steam or electricity, and it does what it is directed to do: it has no power of induction.
>
> Whatever man feels deeply or images clearly, is impressed on the subconscious mind, and carries out in the minutest detail.
>
> For example: a woman I know, when a child, always 'made believe' she was a widow. She 'dressed up' in black clothes and wore a long black veil, and people thought she was very clever and amusing. She grew up and married a man with whom she was deeply in love. In a short time he died and she

wore black and a sweeping veil for many years. The picture
of herself as a widow was impressed on the subconscious
mind, and in due time worked itself out, regardless of the
havoc created.

The conscious mind has been called the mortal or carnal
mind.

It is the human mind and sees life as it *appears to be*. It sees
death, disaster, sickness, poverty and limitation of every
kind, and it impresses the subconscious.

The superconscious mind is the God mind within each
man, and is the realm of perfect ideas.

In it is the 'perfect pattern' spoken of by Plato, The Divine
Design, for there is a Divine Design for each person.

(Florence Scovel-Shinn)

What Florence is saying is that inside us we have an inner self
which, if we allow it, can grow in harmony with God, or the
Divine, and by being in harmony it can create a life for itself
full of health, love and joy.

Luckily for us, the inner movement of our body is always
towards health, and harmony (a cut always tries to heal itself),
but we have to help this movement by not blocking it off with
our negative thoughts and fears. Two simple methods of
encouraging this approach in our mind are affirmations and
visualisations.

The teachers of *rebirthing* are largely responsible for my
learning about affirmations. Sondra Ray describes them beautifully in her book: *I Deserve Love*.

An affirmation is a positive thought that you consciously
choose to immerse in your consciousness to produce a desired
result. In other words, what you do is give your mind an idea
on purpose. Your mind will certainly create whatever you
want it to if you give it a chance. By repetition, you can feed
your mind positive thoughts and achieve your desired goal.

An example of an affirmation is one used by Emile Coué in his
clinic in France at the turn of the century: "Day by day, in every
way, I'm getting better and better."

The Rebirthing movement has developed a more thorough way to use affirmations, but I suggest if you are interested in finding out more you read one of their books. (I include a list at the end of this book of many others you might find of interest.)

Visualisation is a method of first relaxing and then allowing our minds to create certain pictures—a little like conscious day dreaming—to help us heal ourselves. We may spend some time picturing ourselves well, for example; we may picture ourselves in a beautiful environment which makes us feel good.

What we are doing is choosing to give ourselves time in the day when we enter a better space than the one we are in—so that we can draw on the good energies, and draw ourselves towards the better image.

The important thing is to experience how powerful the mind can be, *by doing these things*. It is difficult to believe them without trying them; it is not possible to fully understand them without experiencing them.

> We do not need to believe we can help cure our illness through the power of our positive thoughts. All we need is to want to try. It is experiencing how creative our minds can be that changes our whole perspective.

14

The Mind and Stillness

There was once a merchant. He sold a collection of extremely valuable Genies. One day a man who constantly dreamed of possessing riches and who had scrimped and saved all his life to buy a Genie who would fulfil his every wish, came to the merchant.

"Do you have a Genie to make my dreams come true?" he asked.

"I do" said the merchant and sold it to him. "But be very careful", he warned "if you don't keep the Genie occupied, it will cut off your head."

The man smiled. "Oh I have millions of desires" he said. "I will have no trouble keeping it busy."

No sooner had the man walked a few yards than the Genie bowed and asked: "Task master?"

"Make me a palace, Genie" said the man.
The Genie waved his hand and an enormous and beautiful palace appeared in the distance, at the edge of the town.

"It is done" said the Genie "Task master?"

"That was fast" said the man as he hurried towards his new home "OK, now I want a harem."

Once again the Genie waved his hand and told him it was in the palace waiting for him. "Task master?" the Genie repeated.

"Oh well, a feast, yes I'll have feast in the palace, with every food imaginable waiting for me."

This interplay continued all the way to the place where the man's new home now stood. But by the time they reached the beautiful inner rooms the man was exhausted. He could not eat the food, nor enjoy the pleasure of his harem because the Genie was constantly asking him for his next task.

Eventually the man realised he would never have any peace from the Genie. He was running out of desires and ideas because they were so quickly granted, and he was more and more scared he would lose his head. He ran as fast as he could back to the merchant.

"Please help me", the man begged. "I need some peace."

"I warned you", said the merchant, "but as I am a compassionate man I will tell you what you can do. Tell the Genie to build a tall pole in the garden of your palace and order him to climb up and down this pole until you ask him to stop. Thus you can enjoy the treasures you have wished for."

The man did as he was told and was very grateful.

(Story retold by Chris Jacobs)

This story is about the mind. Our mind is always thinking about something, and needs to be occupied. It is also about meditation: giving the mind something to concentrate on is a way of freeing ourselves from its nagging and giving ourselves time to enjoy the peace and beauty of our inner stillness.

In other words, although our desires (or the man's dreams) may seem real, and our living them out (the Genie) may seem real, and even our fears and worries are real enough, there is a part of us which is none of these things.

The world is perceived, the eyes are its perceiver
The eyes are perceived, the mind is their perceiver
The mind is perceived, the self is its perceiver.

(Ancient Eastern scriptures)

Most of us have realised at one time or another that we are not just our thoughts. We have, as the eastern scriptures say, perceived our minds working, and we know that there is a self, inside us, which is not our minds because it can look at our mind working.

This part of us, our self, sits in our centre, and if we can listen to this part of ourself, we can find a lot of wisdom, or 'inner knowing' right there, waiting for us. Some people call this inner self our inner wise person. Some people think of it as part of our contact with God, or the Divine. Some people even think it is God speaking, and not ourselves at all. Indeed, sometimes the things my inner self says to me are so wise that they don't feel as if they can have come from me, as I know me: sometimes the things my inner self says surprise the rest of me, and I feel that I never knew those things before so how *can* they come just from me?

But this may simply be that I am unable to accept the perfection of my being—or it may be that by coming to my centre I tune into something else, bigger and more profound than my own small personality. I don't know, and it doesn't seem to matter either. Because the important thing is that I—or you—can tune into this centre and find wisdom and healing.

Listening to our centre is not difficult but it does require patience. It requires sitting or lying and allowing the mind to 'turn off' so we can drop into the centre of our being. Luckily for you, sitting and lying is something you are doing a lot of right now, so you don't have to force yourself to get round to starting. You can start any time you please.

Finding the 'calm in the eye of the storm', the serene place inside you, is a pure delight. It's a gift that you'll be giving yourself that can last for the rest of your life. The deepest way to achieve this is through meditation or prayer (and as there are so many good books written on this subject, I won't go on about it myself). If you don't want to follow these options, you may find that simply by sitting and watching the clouds, constantly paying attention to their shape and texture and the play of light on them as they flow across the sky, that you gradually find a peace come over you.

Or again, lying there with your eyes closed, simply spend some time listening to the sound (and feel) of your breath, coming in and going out. Don't be afraid of listening to your breath. (When I first tried it, I was afraid that if I listened I might forget how to breathe, or become so self-conscious that I couldn't breathe, but this turned out to be untrue. I discovered that the breath just goes on *breathing me*, whatever I do or think).

Just keep bringing your attention to the sound of your breath, for no reason, except to listen to your breath. Your mind may start to wander over lots of things (from food, to discomfort, to a new thought...) trying to catch you attention. When this happens, don't be concerned, just smile, and as soon as you find yourself being 'caught' by the thoughts and following them, simply let them go, let them drift away.

Come back again to the sound of your breath. Listen to the wind of it, flowing through you. Listen to its rhythm. After a while of coming back to your breath over and again, you may find your wandering thoughts stop attracting your attention and begin to pass you by, like a stream clattering over tiny pebbles somewhere in the distance, while you feel aware of being in a more 'centred' place in yourself.

This feeling may not be very spectacular, and yet even after as little of fifteen minutes of this, you may feel strangely better in yourself.

> Through the practise of sitting still and following your breath as it goes out and dissolves, you are connecting with your heart. By simply letting yourself be, as you are, you develop genuine sympathy towards yourself.
>
> (*Chogyam Trungpa*)

This is actually a basic meditation technique, and if you want to get the full benefit of it, it is best to sit with your back straight so that you can allow the 'flow of energy' to move up and down your spine.

You can choose what to do with your legs: sitting on a chair means you can have both feet on the ground (the legs should not be crossed), or you can kneel, with support (not too soft or it is uncomfortable) under your bottom. Or you can sit in the eastern meditation position with crossed legs. It is important to be comfortable, and to keep the spine upright. Use a wall to support yourself if necessary.

You don't need to follow any of these 'rules' to get the benefit, and if they put you off, you can explore finding the still place in yourself in whatever way suits you best.

All the meditation techniques (and there are many of them) were created by people who had come to more or less the same truths and wanted to help other people discover them. Therefore they obviously reflect the ideas and character of their creators, and it's up to you to see if any of them suit your personality.

What I like about these techniques is knowing they are created after someone else has gone through a lot of inner searching. They are also part of a long history of knowledge passed—person to person—over the centuries. For those of you who are interested in meditation, I include the words from a leaflet by Ven Lama Sogyal Rinpoche:

Meditation

All our problems come from grasping. Meditation is the means by which we unlearn our tendency to grasp. When we let go, a natural feeling of space arises; this is meditation. Letting go and grasping are both in the mind, this mind which when it is not mindful is so entertainingly, cleverly, sophisticatedly deceptive. Meditation is the path of simplicity, unfolding, adjustment, coming face to face with mind, using mind to tame mind.

The basis of the practice of meditation is relaxation. It is firstly important to be comfortable and allow thoughts and feelings to calm down. There is nothing to attain or achieve, so let go. Let go of any solemnity, and even of the idea that you are meditating. Let your body remain as it is, and breathe as you find it naturally. As for mind, the point is not to suppress thoughts or tail them, but just let them be without being seduced or distracted by them. Do not try to manipulate them. If you are dreaming or thinking...just dream or think...If you do not add fuel, thoughts will just play themselves out.

Gradually things will settle and naturally fall into place. Like pouring a handful of rice onto a flat surface—each grain will settle of its own accord. Once a certain peace of mind is arrived at, straighten your back and alert yourself. Then just let be and continue in relaxation.

If you find it difficult to simply let go and remain so, and you need something to do or follow, be mindful of your breath. If you can not give up activity altogether, then this is skilfully using your activity—to be in tune with yourself.

Each breath is life; simple, powerful, ordinary and free. If you breathe out and don't breathe in again, you are dead. Simply be aware of breath as it comes and goes. One should be lightly mindful and attentive. Be compassionate towards your breath, don't grasp at it or concentrate on it too heavily.

Be with breath, flow with breath. It is as if you are clouds moving across the sky or grasses swayed by the wind. One is simply happening. After you become mindful of breathing for a while, the breath, the breather, and the breathing are one.

When you are no longer conscious of your breath there is a danger of getting stuck in the nowness of breath, becoming unaware. Alert yourself and let go. It is with each breath that we create neurosis, inhibitions, karma. So free yourself with each breath, symbolically, auspiciously, and actually. Be the out-breath; boycott the in-breath. Each breath dissolves into space, suchness, Bhudda nature, or Truth. Then in the space of that spaciousness, almost awestruck, just be. You might never come back!

We start with practice, not perfection: if we were perfect we would not need to practise—"practise makes perfect". We would all like to find the perfect teacher and the perfect practice, rather than make the effort ourselves. So this is a practice and a simple one: breath out—dissolve—space, breath out—dissolve—space. But don't turn it into a mental game or a mechanical exercise and impose a rhythm on it—then there is no space.

For some people, breathing meditation is too close to them, like mind looking at mind naked, so an alternative practice is that of concentration meditation. Rest your mind lightly on an object or image, one which holds positively inspiring and opening associations for you. A flower, a flame—anything that has a feeling of warmth—a sacred image, like one of Buddha or Christ is ideal. Soon you become aware of the suchness of the object, beyond the solid external form. Awareness is no longer differentiating or grasping.

At first practice may be exciting, then boring or even painful. Sit through all these experiences—and even if you can't practise, don't get angry with yourself. Don't think about the practice—just get on with it. Persevere, but with a sense of humour. After a while you will discover a personal style and rhythm. Then you are ready to see a teacher who can advise and guide you in your practice, since there is a shared space of experience. At this point practice is no longer moody or changeable—like British weather—it becomes more spacious. You no longer need technique. You can just be there in the meditative state of mind.

Before attempting to apply meditation in everyday life situations, you should gradually acclimatize to this state of mind. Do not be too adventurous in experimenting with your spiritual strength. Go step by step. Then you can afford to apply it in comfortable, neutral situations, then in unfamiliar situations, then even those of aggression or passion.

With experience of meditation practice, you will develop a skill born of this spaciousness and know when and what to do. Spirituality is not separate from everyday life: the path from practice to enlightenment is through everyday life.

Meditation is neither an instant cure-all that will solve all your problems nor a specific cure for headaches, insomnia etc. It is a gradual process of growth and healing, from it arises the confidence to cope with all life situations.

15

"It's All in the Mind"

Nowadays if an illness cannot be diagnosed, or even if it can but then goes on longer than medical wisdom decrees, it is quite common for doctors (and even alternative practitioners) to say "it's all in the mind".

Unfortunately this phrase implies a criticism of the ill person, or worse, a dismissal of his problems as somehow 'not real'. The same dismissal can be heard in a phrase which is sometimes bandied about the alternative world: 'He doesn't really want to get well' i.e. he is not really trying.

If you have come across this while you are ill, and have found the interference that you should 'pull your socks up' and stop 'imagining things' very upsetting, let me put this to you: perhaps the person who has said this to you has *never been seriously ill*. Why don't you ask them?

It is all too easy for those who have not suffered an ongoing, debilitating illness to make judgements about the way people 'should' behave. They are setting up standards based on ideas (or ideals), or statistics, when they have never had their own particular and individual strengths or weaknesses tested by a painful, depressing situation.

If anyone starts talking to you about things you 'should' or 'ought to' be doing, you may decide to take their advice, but then again you may not. I am always wary of any sentence—including my own—which contains a 'should ' or 'ought'. Those words tell you that someone is making a judgement: and you need to treat it in that way.

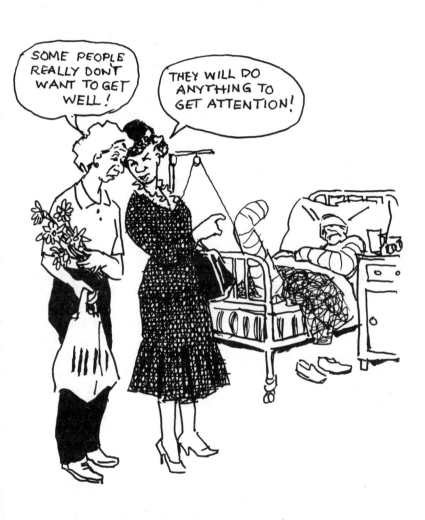

There is no doubt, of course, that our minds are powerful enough to create symptoms in our body just as we can cure ourselves with our minds. Have you ever read about an illness and then found yourself feeling, albeit mildly, some of the symptoms in your body?).

But it can also be *part of our illness* that we get caught in a vicious downward spiral of depression, which is very difficult for our minds to control. (This is why with homeopathic or Bach flower remedies, one of the most encouraging reactions is when we feel 'better in ourselves' even if our symptoms do not immediately disappear). Glandular fever is a good example of an illness which creates chemical changes in the body, producing symptoms of tiredness and depression.

Besides, recognising we can create symptoms with our minds does not make the symptoms any less *real*, because all we are really saying is: one of the terrible and difficult aspects of this illness is that my mind is so distressed that it is creating symptoms *which hurt me*.

Anyone who tells us to 'pull yourself together' rather than showing us compassion for the dilemma in which we are stuck, is trapped in their own 'shoulds and oughts', rather than genuinely trying to help us. Of course if we seem helpless and pathetic, and we carry on as if we were a total victim, our defeatism may well arouse someone's quite natural anger. We would probably feel angry at ourselves too, if we were well.

However, unless we can feel the strength to fight rising up from inside ourselves, other people's words will simply seem like criticisms which only add their weight to the big dark heap which is already weighing us down.

Try not to let their reactions worry you. If you are taking steps to help yourself back to health—with diet, healing, treatment of some sort, some of the exercises at the end of this book, then YOU ARE DOING ALL YOU CAN..

Your energy simply has not caught up with your will to be well.

Give yourself time. Allow whatever needs to unfold a little more attention and space. You never know, this next bit may be the most exciting bit of the whole journey!

16

Listening to More of Yourself

Whether the idea of meditation meant anything to you or not, one thing I hope you began to feel over the last chapters was that your thoughts are not you, only a fascinating and powerful part of you; also that you can use your thoughts to help yourself, and disengage from them when you need to. That, in other words, they are but part of the intricate and marvellous creation into which you woke when you were born on this planet.

Sometimes I think we value our thinking too highly. Within our bodies are other centres of information and wisdom, which function in different ways to thinking, but nevertheless still interpret and interact with life around us. These parts of ourselves work all the time—whether we recognise them working or not—but often we do not listen to them, or we override their information with something we call our 'logic'.

Of course we want to understand our lives to the best of our ability, and act in the most appropriate way—this is why we believe that our minds are the best tools for this purpose.

But what exactly is our mind? Ask someone from Japan or China where their mind is, and they will touch the area below their chest. Ask a child "Whereabouts in your body are you?" and if they don't giggle too much at the question, they will most likely point to their chest or below. They know a difference between mind—which is more like our 'inner knowing', and thoughts—which are more like the computations we make with the information we receive. There is also a difference between thoughts (an idea in response to the moment) and opinions and beliefs (that is fixed ideas arrived at because of past experience and not necessarily relevant to the present situation).

When someone explained to me that my body received information from other areas of myself apart from my head, I found it a very 'freeing' experience. Up until then I had been aware of all sorts of conflicting information coming in at me, but for some reason I had learned not to trust it, rather using my head to try to overrule it. Consequently I ended up doing a lot of things because my thoughts (or beliefs) had decided I should, rather than because I wanted to. In fact I was so bound up in my head, I did not know I was out of touch with the rest of me.

The reason why this is important for me is that I notice that when my 'head runs away with me', I invariably end up ill. If I decide upon an action long before I make it, and blindly follow the *idea,* without checking out whether or not it feels right, whether or not I have enough energy, whether the situation is in fact the one I *thought* it would be, then I am in trouble. In fact, more simply than that, if I lose touch with my centre, I am in trouble. That is why all those 'checks' are part of being 'in balance' and 'in the moment'.

If we look at the English language we can see phrases that express the understanding that other parts of our body have wisdom: 'gut feelings', 'heartfelt desires', 'having our feet on the ground', being 'spineless' and so on. There is nothing esoteric about this, for it is all simple enough. As you read the following descriptions perhaps you would like to stop and 'feel' whether they seem right to you. You may have to rely on as insubstantial a sense as 'they feel vaguely right' or indeed 'they feel vaguely wrong because...'

Your Heart

Take a sentence such as 'Celia agreed with Mr. MacIntyre that she should go on the train to London, but in her heart she knew differently'. What this sentence expresses is: sometimes, no matter how logical an idea is, no matter how completely it convinces our minds, our hearts are also able to make a judgement, which may be different.

Our hearts can tell us one most important thing: whether we are happy, whether the situation we are in (or about to enter) gives us any real joy, or if it can satisfy the longing in our being to be alive and fulfilled, and partaking of a kind of dance with life.

Most of us will have experienced a moment at some time in our life of 'being in love'. This feeling meant that our heart at that time was full of love—and more importantly, we were letting ourselves be in touch with this feeling.

While we are in love the world seems a wonderful place: we skip down the road, and even the smile on the face of the milkman seems to echo the joy we feel inside. We want to run up to people and tell them: the world is a fantastic place!! People seem to us more benevolent and caring. Even when we come across someone who is unhappy, we feel more able to spare them a little of our love—as if we have so much we can afford to! The quality of the day seems more 'alive' to us: light seems brighter, flowers more beautiful, even rain seems something to be enjoyed.

We attach all these feelings or sensations to 'being in love', or, even more commonly, to the actual person we are in love with (it is their smile which makes the sun shine!) But in fact these sensations are not caused by anyone else, but by the fact that we are *in touch with the love energy in our own hearts*. Someone else's love may stimulate the beautiful feeling of love in us, but it is our love, in our hearts, that makes the day brighter for us. (This does not deny, in any sense, the magic of being loved by another). From the love in our hearts comes a special kind of wisdom which has nothing to do with structured logic: this wisdom doesn't *judge* (which is the job of the mind) it understands, it empathises. The heart quality is forgiving simply because, if we feel for another, and listen to their pain—or pleasure—our hearts can empathise with them, rather than want to separate from them and condemn them.

Many books have been written comparing the quality of thought energy: judgement, reason—with heart energy: compassion, nurturing. It seems to be part of our life as human beings that we have to come to some sort of balance between these two aspects, and writers often explore this. Shakespeare does, for example, in the *Merchant of Venice*. Portia pleads with Shylock who wants to extract the exact amount he is due, even if the person he takes it from may die—he appeals to head qualities: logic, rights, laws, and she pleads with him describing heart qualities:

> The quality of mercy is not strained
> It droppeth as the gentle rain from heaven
> upon the place beneath
> It is twice blessed: it blesseth him
> that gives and him that takes...

Portia is saying that a gesture from the heart makes us feel good as well as the person to whom we give. She is also trying to stir with the 'heart quality' of her words, the same quality in Shylock.

A human being needs to be able to measure and judge things in order not to be swamped by the outside world, to be able to order, and contain. Equally she needs to be able to go beyond boundaries, to listen to movement within her, and within another, and respond, in order to create happiness, well-being, joy.

The important thing is that 'being in love' is not the only way to experience this awakening to the beauty of life through our hearts. We do not need to have anyone else to 'attach' this love to. Moreover if we are in touch with our hearts, the feeling of love is there awaiting us, no matter what our external situation is. While love is the primary emotion in our hearts, we also have there: pain, grief, despair, hurt. When we begin to open to our heart area, it is sometimes difficult to feel the love, because our hearts are so full of these other feelings. But if we can bear to listen to these other feelings too, and deal with them, we will find an inner compassion for ourselves, and that compassion will lead us to love.

Suffering and hurt and pain are doorways: we either slam the door shut and try to keep it all away from us—so that our lives become dry and arid, our hearts closed from us, and our whole body tensed in the effort to keep it that way; or we open the door and as we do so, so our hearts open too, and we can feel again, not only for ourselves, but for others.

> I have a friend, a chemotherapy nurse in a children's cancer ward, whose job it is to pry for any available vein in an often emaciated arm to give infusions of chemicals that sometimes last as long as twelve hours, and which are often quite discomforting to the child. He is probably the greatest pain giver the children meet in their stay in hospital. Because he has worked so much with his own pain, his heart is very open. He works with his responsibilities in the hospital as a 'laying on of hands with love and acceptance'. There is little in him that causes him to withdraw, that reinforces the painfulness of the experience for the children. He is a warm open space which encourages them to trust whatever they feel. And it is he whom the children most often ask for when they are dying. Although he is the main pain giver, he is also the main love giver.
>
> (Ram Dass & Paul Gorman: *How Can I Help?*)

The area of the heart fills the whole of the bottom of the rib cage, and although it reaches the chest or the breasts, it can be more deeply felt further back.

Your Solar Plexus

The solar plexus is the area in the centre of our trunk, just below the front of the rib cage, and above the tummy button. Again, when getting in touch with the area, remember to go in deep and back. The American Indians say we have a cord going from here to the Great Spirit.

The solar plexus is the area of our body which squeezes up like mad whenever we have a sudden shock: for instance we are driving along the road and suddenly we just miss having a serious accident. The feeling of sudden shock is like a sudden punch in our stomach. This gives us a clue about one way our solar plexus works: it is our detector of tension and danger. It tells us whether we are in a situation that is about to hurt us or knock us 'off balance'.

Underneath our solar plexus is what I call our **will**. The will is our ability to feel whole and strong, to carry out an action in a way that keeps us whole, strong and centred. Most people living in Western cultures have lost touch with this part of their body. Learning to be in touch with it and move from it is central to most martial arts. The understanding is that from the solar plexus to the bottom of the pelvis is the area of strength of our body, and the centre of our balance.

If we consider ourselves in this way: our chest and head, our legs and arms are all spokes coming out of this central hub of ourselves. This thought allows us to move these 'outer' parts of ourselves like the rim of the wheel, and still keep our weight or our 'being' in our central hub, so that we don't get caught off balance.

> The solar plexus is the spiritual/psychic 'brain' of Man, the confluence of Cosmic and Earthly forces, the blender and balancer of opposite influences, and the centre of the physical and spiritual umbilical cord. Earth energy is drawn up via the feet, and Cosmic energy is drawn down via the head, meeting in the solar plexus (or 'Tan t'ien').
>
> (Beverley Milne: *Tai Chi, spirit and essence.*)

Without straying into the intricacies of Tai-chi and other martial arts, it is simply interesting for you to understand that if ever you felt you were wound up, off balance, knocked about by people and events, weak-willed and unable to achieve what you had set out to achieve, that what you were feeling was out of touch with this part of yourself.

If you close your eyes now and examine this area of yourself, you may only be able to feel something like a knot of tension, or a sensation of tightness—which might make you feel anxious, or 'unpleasant'. Your solar plexus is registering the amount of tension in your body—but this may not be simply present tension, but stored from years of tightening in that area.

Don't worry if you find it difficult to stay in contact. Be patient. Begin gently to breathe into that area: imagine your breath like gentle strokes of wind, unwinding the many skeins and threads of the knot, slowly and gently. The solar plexus also registers other people in a different way to our mind. It is as if we have 'feelers' coming out of that area of ourselves which 'sense' other people.

Maybe you can remember speaking to someone once and feeling a sudden knotting up of that area. It was your way of letting yourself know you were in danger. The other person, no matter how nice they seemed, logically, had some kind of negative effect on you.

This kind of information or 'wisdom' is very useful to us once we are in touch with it. When we feel this squeeze in the presence of someone, it doesn't mean they are necessarily a bad person at all: it may mean we are letting ourselves be manipulated by them. (People 'good and bad' may manipulate each other.) It may mean we are acting with them in a way we really feel awkward or unhappy about—or that we are letting their presence make us 'off-balance'. It may also mean we are panicking in their presence: we might experience this feeling in a job interview, or even on seeing a policeman approach us. It is a signal for us to watch out, to take care; to remember to breathe and stay in touch with our area of strength.

Your Hara

The hara occupies the lower space, below the tummy button, to the base of the pelvis.

During a good healing session we are most likely to experience a sensation of 'dropping down' into the lower parts of ourselves. Accompanying this feeling of 'dropping' down' is a sense of stillness and strength.

If we look at a picture of the spine we can see that the thickest and strongest vertebra are between the bottom of our rib cage down to the inside of our pelvis—and the pelvic bowl itself is largest area of bone in the whole body. What this tells us is that this area was designed by nature to *carry weight*. In other words it is in real structural terms an area of support and strength for us. Being able to be *in* this space in ourselves is the best way to feel strong and at ease. The feeling of inner strength is nothing like a mental decision to feel strong—it is an actual bodily sensation, coming from the fact that we are using our body as it was designed.

Thoughts and emotions can cause us great turbulence, stress, and upset *if we get stuck in them*; that is if we live only in the top quarter of our bodies. The hara area is our way to freedom. We can't think our way out of our thoughts, or feel our way out of our feelings, but we *can* experience being in the centre of ourselves, and feeling calm because we are no longer caught 'up' in our heads or hearts only. You may have difficulty imagining this: but if you are lucky enough to find a healer or an experience which lets you see this, it will make absolute sense.

The hara area is one of the most forgotten in our Western culture: even our dancing involves more movement of head and shoulders than it does of the belly and pelvis! This is in part because although we are bombarded with stories and movies about sex, and page three girls (perhaps *because* we are bombarded by them) for most of us our own sexuality causes us quite a bit of embarrassment and tension. The hara area contains not only our sexual organs, but out reproductive systems: ovaries, gonads, and our eliminative systems: another source of embarrassment and tension for us.

Few people breathe right down into their pelvic areas and most people (quite unconsciously) keep their pelvic floor muscles squeezed in a chronic state of tension. Most of us seem to be constantly trying to 'pull away' from our more animal selves, towards our heads, or even spirits. But of course we can't *really* pull away from ourselves; all we can do is to lose touch with half of our body and over-emphasise the other half (or quarter). As appealing as this might be to our heads, if nature had intended it this way, she would have designed us differently. Besides, sexuality is a wonderful gift, and is important to our health: not the sexual act itself, but a lively, awake awareness of the sensual nature of our bodies.

In our culture we seem to suffer a lot of confusion about the word sexuality: we tend to think of it as only what we call 'making love', and by that we really mean the sexual act of penetration. Included in our idea of sexuality is: abuse, rape and aggression. People still talk about rape as if it were a sexual act, rather than what it really is: an act of violence.

Sensuality is something we seem to ignore quite a bit when we talk of sexuality. Sensuality is an awakeness to the beauty and feel of the other: the touch of a leaf, the feel of skin, the warmth of a smile, the sensation of a warm rug under bare feet.

We cannot be open to the vibrant, stimulating, sensual beauty of the world around us without involving our own sexual natures in our appreciation of life. Once again, this does not mean copulation, but it does mean allowing an inner movement, a flow, an interaction.

Life has given us this wonderful gift of a sexual response, and the gift of free will, so that we can choose how much or how little of this response to display at any given moment. If we are going to accept that we are worthy of love and healing, we are also going to accept that we are worthy of pleasure.

No doubt if you are very ill, you hardly want to think about your sexuality at the moment, and indeed, too much sexual stimulation can be very draining while our energy levels are low. But breathing into your pelvic area will bring about a sense of well-being that is vaguely sensual in nature, and it is important not to feel guilty or worried about this, or to feel you have any need to turn it into a full blown sexual feeling either!

The wisdom of our hara area is the wisdom of our raw, basic instincts. When we talk about our 'gut reaction' we may sometimes be talking about our solar plexus reaction, but more often it is something we call our instincts. 'Instincts' are unqualified, unjustified reactions. We can have an instinct and then later on work out reasons to justify it, but it is a much quicker reaction that thought.

Some people in touch with their 'instincts' would argue that they are very rarely wrong. They can be a sort of inner knowing, which picks up all sorts of signs and signals our brains ignore, and which doesn't need to understand why it knows. These instincts are part of, but not quite the same as intuition. A person who uses his intuition is someone who can stay in the quiet centred part of himself and listen both to his instincts, and to his heart.

Intuition is full of heart in that it is concerned with what feels right and good, whereas instinct feeling is more basic, it is concerned with survival, pleasure, raw truth; such as the truth of a small child: "Mummy, I don't like that man, he looks mean".

As we grow more sophisticated we learn to override these instinctual truths. In many cases this is necessary and good—we don't want to withdraw from someone simply because we don't find his face attractive—but we can begin to override them to such an extent that we are no longer aware what our true basic reactions are.

When they are suppressed to such an extent, our instincts then tend to rush out in huge uncontrollable bursts at odd moments—most of us know of 'nice', 'quiet' people who get drunk and behave 'outrageously ', perhaps even going off with someone we think is quite 'unsuitable' for them. (Perhaps you recognise some aspect of this in yourself.)

This behaviour leads to a vicious circle: in the morning, overcome with shame and guilt we suppress our instincts even more strongly; because they are so suppressed, the next time they surface with an uncontrollable force again; this makes us dislike them and feel afraid of them, pushing them down again.

To escape this cycle we again need to use our solar plexus—or centre—or wise self. Just as we can't escape mind with mind—we can't escape instinct with instinct. But we can begin to open to this aspect of ourselves, begin to appreciate its use to us, and allow it to feed and nourish our relationships with the world, while using our hearts and minds to ensure it acts in a more responsible manner. (More on this in Chapter 21)

Your Feet

By far the wisest parts of our body are our feet. Noticing whether our feet are in touch with the ground is an immediate barometer which tells us whether or not we are 'letting our minds run away with us' or if we are 'grounded'.

Though we can't listen to our feet in the same way as our other centres, we can observe them. Simply noticing whether the skin underneath our heel, down each outside of our arches, underneath the top pad of the foot, and underneath the toes is in contact with the floor or ground. If the contact feels 'screwed-up' or 'shaky' or 'tight' this gives us information about ourselves too.

Suppose we think we are 'on top of the world' and yet when we observe our feet—the part of us which actually contacts the top of the world—we notice that they feel 'light', out of contact, a bit 'shaky', doesn't that tell us something interesting?

Our toes have the best sense of humour of any part of our body. If you want to smile: just wriggle your toes. If you try having a conversation with your toes, you may even laugh.

One of the things which is clear when we consider our other centres is how much they are to do with caring for us, looking after our well-being.

An important part of regaining our health is learning to trust and rely on 'other' information that comes our way. Our brain is sometimes quite resistant to being pushed off its throne; it insists it is the only voice worth listening to. Our brain will create a lot of good arguments against listening to anything but its logic.

One of them is: it's not safe. We think that if we are not mentally in control we risk spinning off into an unknown zone of catastrophe and darkness. We may be tossed about by our feelings, dragged along by our instincts. But our brain is not safe either. We have already realised the way our thoughts can keep us in a state of frustration by having us chase impossible ideals.

Our ability to reason and dissect is important, but if it runs counter to our feelings, or our deepest instincts, to continue following it is to invite breakdown. Our system cannot cope with the various parts tugging against each other. The design is so simple: each centre adding to the wisdom of the other so that we can partake of life in a healthy, productive way.

Out thoughts may try to reason away other aspects of our being—our feelings, our instincts—but of course it is impossible to do so. We can't reason away something which is part of ourselves—we can only fool ourselves into thinking we have! By learning to listen to other parts we don't deny our brain, on the contrary we use its fantastic skill in listening and interpreting the signals.

Picture your body as a circle. In the centre is you; and your wise self. Around the circle we put: thoughts, feelings, will and instincts.

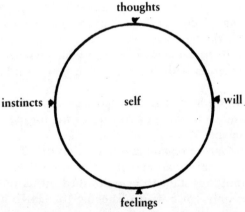

Each of the outer centres can feed your inner self. Similarly you can listen to, and nurture your outer centres. In this way you can benefit from all that your being can give you, and in return your being can feel appreciated and loved.

The way I have described our centres makes it appear as if I know exactly where everything is, when of course I don't. What I have written is to try to help you explore yourself, but there is no reason for you to trust any of it unless it feels true to you.

What is important is: that you being to trust two things: that your wisdom is far greater than the wisdom of your brain, and that you are just as able as I am to start listening to yourself.

Indeed you are far more able to listen to yourself than I am able to listen to you! You know all the ins and outs of your life: you know your desires, your fears, your limits, your abilities far better than anyone else. And you are also the only one able to find people to help you, if you need it.

So how can you set about listening to yourself? First of all listening is *not* imagining in your head what these parts of yourself would or should say. They may not speak in clear language, it might seem a bit nebulous at first.

Is there a clock in your room, or anything outside the room making a regular sound? Take a few minutes and listen to it. Allow your breath to release, so that air can come in again. Keep your awareness on releasing your breath. Relax. Don't overconcentrate on the noise: notice if you are tightening any part of your body (in particular your neck or jaw or shoulders) in order to 'hear'. If so, let them relax. Keep paying attention to releasing your breath. Do not try to 'grab onto' the sound, but observe the quality and flavour of the tick by relaxing and letting the sounds come to you.

This is one way to listen. When you apply it to listening to parts of yourself, remember you are listening to something as real and substantial as the ticking of the clock.

17

Emotion

Emotions can have a very strong effect on us: we can 'see with anger', 'tremble with frustration', and of course 'cry with sorrow'. And there are also other emotions, consider the phrase: 'eaten up with resentment' or again 'twisted with bitterness'. These phrases vividly describe the effect a long term, stored up emotion can have on us—anything unresolved and unloved in us can take its toll on our being.

As human beings we feel a range of feelings every day and we are unlikely to recognise them all, or sort them all out. Besides it often feels too painful or two difficult to come to terms with things that happen to us in the past, and in order to get on with our lives now, we tend to push those things aside.

It may be, though, that when you started listening to yourself you became aware of some quite strong emotions which seemed to rise up from inside you, and perhaps make it difficult for you to go on listening. Many painful feelings come from hurt and loss. Someone did not love us as we loved them; a parent died; a partner left us. At the time we may have been overwhelmed by sadness, but because we had to go on living we eventually pushed the pain aside. We tried to leave it behind, but somehow the pain never quite left us.

Many people manage to ignore their pain for a long time—some, I suppose, forever. But many others suffer an illness sometime in the future—as if the running away has to come to a stop. I am not saying that all illness is caused by past grief, but because we are a whole organism, our feelings are as important for our recovery as any other part of our being. Some griefs can still hurt us so badly that we have to become ill to really see them, to realise they are there, and hopefully, to come to terms with them. This does not mean that we sort them out, or change the past, or solve them. Some things have no solution. Perhaps because of this we avoid looking at the problem: the pain. Coming to terms with a problem does not mean solving it, although something might be solved in the process.

If something happened to you which still hurts, you might like briefly to consider your life since the event. Do you feel that part of you was running away from the depth of hurt and despair you felt? Were any of your daily actions a way of trying to compensate, or cover up? The main feeling to notice is one of being driven, and yet of avoiding something by driving so fast; of a despair that seemed to haunt you, that you were afraid of falling into.

Before I was ill last time I had been putting a lot of energy into achieving a particular ambition. All seemed to be going well, and I became blind to the many problems because I wanted it so much. Only after I became ill and had to let my ambition go did I realise why I wanted it so much; my wanting clouded my judgement because I had fixed on it as a way of forgetting my past loss.

The reason I was so desperate for the ambition not to fail was because when it did I was left with seeing what I was running away from. Yet the driving power behind my ambition—in all honesty—was not so much to fulfil myself as to prove to someone else that I was alright (very alright) without him.

When people go they do not take that time in *your* life with them. That piece of the past is still yours: yours to love or be angry about, yours to treasure or forget.

The memory does not even have to be good, to be honoured as *important to you*. Perhaps your parents have died or left, and you found your relationship with them difficult; nevertheless you loved them perhaps in some way they had deep meaning in your life, and that is part of your past. People often talk about not getting stuck in the past. And it is true that it is not healthy for us to live only in the past.

But carefully here: we can say the same about being ill. We might not want to go on being ill. We might not want to go on being affected by our past, but we *are* still affected. We don't know why this is so—but it is. Either we can deny the truth and start running again as soon as we are able, or we can say: "Well it seems I am even more affected by this than I realised. Obviously there is more mourning to be done. There is more to be honoured, more to be healed."

We can't live our life without a past, any more than a building can exist without its foundations. We don't need to dwell in the past, or identify with it, but we can't deny that the past happens, or that it affected the person we are today.

Sometimes the decision to accept we are still hurting, can feel like an enormous relief:

> As long as I was pushing away the pain, it had me nailed to the wall. But then I stopped resisting it. I sort of let it in. It was actually a relief. I felt better in spite of it. No longer at odds with everything.
>
> (Ram Dass & Paul Gorman: *How Can I Help?*)

If we run away from something, the irony is that we are not free of it at all: our very avoidance *is* the motor which drives us on. We are still caught up in the pain, even if we spend our time refusing to have the pain. And our lives are ruled by the past hurt much more than they would be if we simply gave up running and wept.

If, when you start to breathe into your body, feelings do come up for you, they may well be part of your illness, and facing them part of your cure. If you find this hard to accept: remember people do *die* of a broken heart. Grief and pain can have a powerful, depleting effect on our systems.

One thing seems relevant here: in our society we seem to have a time limit on how long we can be sad about losing someone. (And about where and when it is appropriate to be sad). We can weep for a week, mourn for a few more, and then it is no longer easy to express to others how much sadness and confusion still lingers. This is particularly true if we split up with someone—when he (or she) is gone, he is every bit as gone, to us, as if he were dead, but we suffer the rejection as well as the loss. Meanwhile there is a subtle pressure which says: you should be over this and on to pastures new!

Mourning someone who is gone (whether she is dead or departed) is a way of *honouring* her, and all the beautiful things that happened with her. The honouring of what you have lost is nothing to be ashamed of—there is no reason why you should not remember the things which made you love your loved one, or why you should not remember the times you had together, the places you saw together. When we push our pain 'away' where do you imagine it goes? When we feel upset but 'keep the feeling down' what happens to the feeling? Does it disappear? Emotions are energy forms and they don't go away: they can be changed, but they don't just go.

When you work with a person's body, it seems that emotions can actually be stored in his tissue and muscle. If you stroke or massage tissue in a certain way, feelings actually 'come up' for people—literally as if they had been released from the body and moved upwards.

If feelings are 'kept down' they are kept down in the musculature and tissue of our body. Imagine the effect over time of a feeling of anger, or resentment boiling inside us!

The ironical thing about life is that while most of us recognise that spoken anger and bitterness can hurt other people, we are loath to recognise that stored up anger and bitterness can harm ourselves. And not only harm us emotionally, but actually attack our body tissue as well. The most destructive emotions to store are bitterness, resentment, and guilt; these are poisonous, creeping emotions which stay inside us and literally eat away at our systems. It is vital if you feel any of these emotions about past events in your life, to deal with them and let them go. You have to allow forgiveness for yourself and others. Forgiveness lets in love. And love heals. You may find it hard to forgive someone who has hurt you badly, you may feel they don't deserve your good feelings. But remember you are doing this for *your* sake, not their's. You want your being to be filled with love, not with poisonous emotions, don't you? When we push one strong feeling down, we can only do it by pushing down all our feelings—the good ones as well as the bad.

If we push away our hurt and pain, we reject our ability to love and care for ourselves, in fact if we do this too often or too strongly we may deny all feeling. We start to feel numb inside. We are aware, perhaps, of a dull build-up of depression which seems to threaten us. We try to avoid it. Sometimes our avoidance can be one of the reasons we work so hard and make ourselves ill. (As if we can't truly avoid something— because when we are ill we have so much time for such things to stare us in the face.)

If we can turn and face our feelings of pain, we can find our feelings of love as well. But this is not something you can suddenly decide to do—it may well be you need to turn to someone for help. Do you have a friend to talk to? Can you tell your practitioner? (Most practitioners would like to know how you are feeling, because they understand that this is all part of your getting well. You don't have to justify your need. Perhaps if you need to cry, you could consider just crying without even saying why—if you don't feel up to sharing it with words, just share the feelings.

If you do want to listen on your own, in a gentle, caring way: make sure you create a safe environment for yourself —invite a friend or neighbour to call or to stay. Have someone to phone if you need to. (You can always phone the Samaritans or some crisis centre). Then allow yourself to feel a little bit more, a bit deeper than before. This does *not* mean that you decide you are going to experience a set of feelings and set about reproducing them. Nor does it mean to stir yourself up unnecessarily. You are aiming to be *in touch* with your feelings, not to solve them. Don't push yourself: your real feelings will reveal themselves as soon as you approach them with love.

Don't expect you will suddenly find a 'repressed' feeling

and—lo and behold—once you have released it you will be miraculously cured. (It's always possible this may happen, I suppose). This process of listening to our feelings is not so much about getting them out—because that can be merely another way of trying to be rid of them—as learning to accept how we are feeling at any given time. We can then go on in one whole piece, and take our feelings 'into account'.

Often when we tune into our feelings they don't turn out to be as noble or profound as we had hoped. Often when I tune into myself I find a rather small someone saying 'help'. This person is often so afraid she longs for someone else to *live her life for her*. 'I am being brave and positive, while this part of me just wants to give up and weep.'

Giving yourself a chance to express your feelings doesn't mean the outer problem will be solved. For instance weeping can't return a lost loved one. Hearing your despair because you are so fed up being ill, won't make you well. But weeping or hearing your despair can help you to face up to your human condition: to realise your neediness, to realise your vulnerability, *and to find a part of yourself that cares about you*, and an inner strength which is able to choose to go on living, knowing your vulnerability and need.

> To know you are vulnerable does not make you a victim.
> To know you feel helpless does not make you beaten
> For one so weak to go on living is a sign of real strength.

Finding the part of yourself can sympathise with all you are going through is a wonderful thing. Remember to make yourself comfortable. Remember to keep yourself warm. Stroke your own brow. Tell yourself 'It's alright, I love you'.

> I tell myself 'I love you' most days now. I've learnt to recognise times when I am feeling a bit down and could do with some attention. I also try to remember to encourage myself. It never makes me feel 'puffed up'—on the contrary it helps me realise how needy I am, and how grateful I am to myself, for a bit of attention.
>
> (Conversation with a friend)

You do not have to go through life feeling scared of yourself, or ignoring something precious in the hope it will go away. If there is a part of you that feels sad, you deserve comfort. If you daren't ask your friends for comfort, if you don't know how to begin to comfort yourself—go and see a healer, a teacher, counsellor or therapist who will help you.

It is such a lovely feeling receiving care from someone else. Especially as many of the hurts we have suffered in life have been at the hands of someone else—it is wonderful to allow another person to heal those hurts.

For example, suppose you are someone whose mother misunderstood or mistreated you in some way: it is wonderful to be able to let yourself be 'mothered' by a woman who is a healer. She won't be your mother, of course, but you can allow her voice, her touch, her care, to soothe some of your hurts, and from her you can learn how to treat yourself with care. Or suppose you have been raped or sexually abused by a man. To allow yourself to build up a relationship of trust with a man who is a healer, to allow your body to receive his care—is to give yourself a chance to soothe away the shock, to 'wash-clean' and start again.

A remarkable thing in this life is that people can heal each other. Your healer/teacher may (will probably) be only a person with as many problems as you have, and yet, because of the quality of their attention and care, you can be helped by them. Because you gradually begin to trust them, you begin to trust yourself.

The fact that human beings can do this for each other saves us from drifting further into our own pain and destruction—it gives us hope for our future, for everyone's future. It is a wonderful thing!

Allow yourself to be helped by this precious truth about life. Somewhere out there is someone who can help you. If you have read this book this far, you are certainly quite capable of finding them.

18

Listening to Your Pain

Good food adequate rest, warmth and something to make us laugh are basic to getting well. Periods of mental calm, times of thinking positively are important. Learning to listen to our needs, starting to care for ourselves, is perhaps the most important thing of all—especially in the long run. I don't mean to dwell on pain, but I would like you to read this chapter as part of the whole process of getting well—indeed I imagine each chapter as a little mirror, each part of a bigger mosaic of mirrors, reflecting the many intricacies of illness.

We can use the understanding that feelings do not just disappear when we ignore them, but stay buried within us, possibly within our very body tissue, to help us understand our pain.

In a little booklet, '*Heal your body*—The mental causes for physical illness and the metaphysical way to overcome them' the author, Louise L Hay explains that the very places *where* our bodies choose to hurt, and the very *kind* of hurting we feel, carry an important message for us. For example, if my throat is sore, this tells me that I have pain in the area of speaking/communicating. Perhaps there was something I wanted to say but didn't—something, in other words, I buried in my throat, which is now hoarse and hurting.

Another example is sinus trouble—this is about held back anger, something inflammatory which we held back. I found this concept very useful: several years ago I used to have sinus trouble quite badly and fairly regularly. Now I don't have it at all (though occasionally a dull ache gives me a little warning to pay attention). I cured this firstly by learning to take simple measures to care for my sinuses—like not taking too many 'mucus forming' foods, and keeping them warm in cold weather. I also learned that whenever they started to ache was a sign for me to find out what I was stewing over, and to 'spit it out' so that the anger (inflammation) didn't build up.

Quite recently a friend of mine was due to go abroad on holiday. She was very excited, but also very nervous. Just before she went, her left hip gave way and she was in agony. It lasted one evening, when she gave herself a lot of care and attention, and the hip reverted to normal. Translated, it was her way of saying: 'I am scared of moving forward, I am scared of stepping out into the unknown'.

The same thing happened to a friend of mine who was a climber. He came to visit me on his way to Russia, where he was due to do a very difficult climb as part of an American team. For no apparent reason he suddenly got a very bad and stiff neck, causing him excrutiating pain. This went of its own accord by the time he got to Russia, where he was, indeed, about to risk his neck.

I include a brief list of some of the connections here, but for a more comprehensive list, please get hold of the booklet I have taken them from. Louise Hay also lists some positive or new thought patterns that can help.

Problem	Probable Cause	New thought Pattern
Addictions	Self-rejection, fear, lack of love	I am only addicted to loving myself. Nothing has power over me.

Problem	Probable cause	New thought pattern
Back problems	Lack of support *Upper*: Lack of emotional support. *Lower*: Lack of financial support. Fear of money.	Life itself supports me. I trust the Universe. I freely give love and trust.
Bronchitis	Inflamed family environment.	Peace. No one can irritate me.
Constipation.	Refusing to release old ideas. Stinginess.	I release the past. I generously allow life to flow through me.
Eye problems	Not liking what you see in your own life. Fear of the future. Fear of the Truth.	I see with loving eyes. I like what I see, I see clearly. I see the Truth.
Heart problems	Serious emotional problems of long standing. Lack of joy, rejection of life. Belief in strain and pressure.	Joy, joy, joy. Love and peace. I joyfully accept all of life.
Holding fluids	What you are afraid of losing.	I release with joy and willingness.
Indigestion	Fear, dread, anxiety.	I take in the new and easily assimilate it.
Kidney problems	Criticism, sensitivity, disappointment, frustration.	I see only good everywhere. Right action is taking place and I am fulfilled.

Problem	Probable Cause	New thought Pattern
Leg problems	Fear of the future, Legs carry you forward.	I move forward with confidence and joy.
Liver problems	Depression. Repression. Chronic complaints. Liver is the seat of anger.	I live life through the open space in my heart. I am free to love.
Neck	Inflexibility, refusing to see all sides of a question. Stubborn.	I am flexible, I welcome other viewpoints too.
Slipped disc	Indecision. Not feeling emotionally supported by others.	I am courageous and independent. I am supported by life.
Ulcers	Something eating away at you. Anxiety, fear tension. Belief in pressure.	Nothing can irritate me. I am peaceful, calm and at ease.

I did not include this list to make you feel more self-critical, or more anxious or worried. It is only a little help to realise your illness is in part caused by anxiety, if you are already feeling anxious. We cannot manufacture a feeling of peace and serenity out of nowhere! Instead of looking at our illness as if it is something quite alien to us, quite unconnected to our lives, these associations help us build a picture which shows us that our illness is an expression of ourselves, and of the difficulties we are facing in our life. Because the illness is an expression of ourselves, contained within the kind of pain we have, it is a clue to help us to see how we can help ourselves, but not to find extra things to worry about!

. There are other ways you can listen to the message your pain is giving you. Listen to the tone or quality of the hurting:

it is inflamed, sore, aching, sharp? Inflammation can be to do with anger—either too much expression of it to no end, or a holding back of it, or an ongoing feeling of it bubbling inside.

Soreness— what kind is it? An angry soreness? An irritated, frustrated soreness? A weeping soreness? When you listen, take note of how the pain makes you feel, that may help you discover the feeling of the pain. For example, suppose listening to it makes you feel sad and helpless. Perhaps the quality of the pain is a weeping quality. It hurts as if it were clinging to you.

Aching—is it an aching like sadness—like heartache—of sorrow and loss, or is it an aching like bitterness, like resentment, a feeling of being cheated? Does it make you want to curl up and be still, does it make you want to rant and rave? If it is sharp—does it beat you down? Does it needle you? Does it make you cringe and gasp? It is hot? Does it make you crease up? Do you feel skewered on it?

If we are in pain it is often very difficult for us to keep our concentration on the area of ourselves that hurts. Our desire is to pull away, to make the same flinching movement we make when we burn a finger—pull back, try to shake it off, to stop the hurting. Whatever you do, don't make listening to your pain a battle. Don't feel you have to grit you teeth and dive in there—through the wall of flames—desperately trying to protect yourself from the burning heat.

To begin to notice a few things about your pain, don't push too hard. Let yourself nip quickly into the area, notice for a second, and come back. Or lie and let the feeling or sensation come to you, observe it lightly, but don't linger on it.

It is important for us to be patient. We can grow more familiar with our pain if we give ourselves a little time. But it is not a competition or a struggle. Hearing ourselves is an act of love. Remember this each time: hearing ourselves is an act of love. We only listen because we want to heal. Don't try too hard to work anything out. In fact it is far better if you use your mind to avoid working anything out. Keep consciously doing this, and perhaps a thought might come to you.

You might want to put your hand (if you can) over the area of the pain—about an inch above it, and gently stroke, either as you would a cat, or in a gentle circular motion, depending on whichever feels right. (Clockwise draws energy in, anti-clockwise sends energy out). First and foremost, begin to let your pain know you care about it. Begin to let yourself know you care about your pain.

Listening to our pain is not easy: and very often we don't get a clear message. This is important: your pain most probably *won't* say: 'I am hurting because you didn't tell your mother that you love her' or some such sage advice. Also it won't say: 'I'm hurting because you didn't take that holiday you needed'. You might want to blame yourself and look for a hook on which to hang your blame—but although the pain may be hurt or angry, it won't be full of *blame*, in the sense of blaming you. If only it was that simple! Find out what we did wrong, tell ourselves off, say sorry, and woosh...away goes the pain!!!

When you practise listening to your pain, try to remain honest to yourself if you are not feeling anything. Don't be tempted by an idea. Often we can listen for five to ten minutes with no clear image at all, and then something very insignific-ant flashes into our thoughts or feelings. But if we learn to trust it—no matter how small it is—we are beginning to 'hear'.

Let me give you an example: Jane is listening to her pain. She feels resentful that the pain has come back again and finds it hard really to pay it attention with an open heart. Her mind keeps wandering. She notices that all she wants is for the pain to be gone. She does not want to hear it. She thinks: 'Perhaps there's something I don't want to hear'. She doesn't try to follow the idea, but puts it to one side. But the idea has made her interested in listening further.

The pain hurts. She can feel it hurting in all sorts of different areas, and as she follows it, it seems to change from moment to moment. She can't define its texture at all, except that it is unpleasant to stay with the pain. It seems if she keeps noticing it, it becomes worse and worse. She feels the pain becoming 'loud', but she can't attach an emotion to it.

She decides to try to follow the pain to its centre, to the place where the pain is at the worst. She suddenly remembers to notice her breathing, and consciously to breathe air into the area in pain. She discovers the first area she noticed does not seem to be where the pain is coming from. It seems to be further back, more difficult to get to. She thinks: 'it feels twisted'. As she thinks that the pain seems to spin in her mind and untwist, then settle in one place. It makes her feel sad. Then she finds her concentration is wandering: she's been thinking about something else for the last few seconds. She decides to breathe healing into the area and then stop.

I use this example precisely because nothing spectacular happened. Obviously your experience won't be like Jane's: more or less may happen. What Jane immediately got out of this experience was two thoughts: That she was in some state she didn't want to hear, and something was twisted, and when it untwisted she felt sad. She may want to pay further attention to this—particularly if she can connect it to some event or feeling. But she doesn't need to. If Jane leaves this alone, the chances are that because she has started a process by listening, something may come to her later on anyway.

In this particular case Jane *did* feel sad about something some time later. Although she could try to 'buck herself up' she chooses instead to let herself cry. She is surprised to find out how much she wants to cry. She feels sorry for herself. She discovers she was saddened by something one of her visitors said. Although he may not have meant it that way, it touched on an inner fear she had, and made her feel it quite painfully. Jane now comforts herself or—if she is able—sorts out the hurt with the visitor. Amazingly the pain seems to subside.

This does not mean that all pain will go as soon as we recognise it and 'sort something out'. If only it would! But at least if we begin to sort things out as they happen, we are not adding to our condition, and we are learning a way of being in touch with ourselves which could help us all our lives. And of course there is always the chance the pain *will* be helped too.

Questioner: How can I be sure that I am seeing what to do?
Krishnamurti: You can't see what to do, you can only see what not to do. The total negation of that road is the new beginning, the other road. The other road is not on the map, nor can it ever be put on any map. Every map is a map of the wrong road, the old road.

(Krishnamurti, from *Don't push the River* by B. Stevens)

The Dialogue

Of course, pain does not have vocal cords, so it cannot have a voice as we understand it ordinarily. Anything we picture, feel, vaguely hear in our heads, could be connected to our pain *once we have instructed our minds to focus on it.*

Obviously we need to focus our minds on the question, or area of enquiry, before we can expect anything we observe to be relevant. When we begin, it is necessary:

To approach our pain with love,

To focus on our pain with our minds,

Once we have done this, a third thing is also necessary:

To trust that everything is of value.

We begin as usual by allowing ourselves to relax—probably lying down. Gently move your thoughts around your body encouraging each part of yourself: feet, legs, bottom, hips, back, arms, shoulders, neck, head, jaw, to relax and soften. Notice your breathing: allowing the breath to come into your body, down your spine, as far as you can imagine into your pelvis, before letting it travel up again and out.

Imagine that along with air, you are breathing in light, something like soft sunlight, gentle and soothing, and full of healing. Keep breathing this light into yourself as you move in your mind over to the part of yourself in pain. Come to your pain, breathing light and healing as you approach, so that you can imagine your attention healing yourself even as you listen.

Observe the 'quality' of pain. Notice if any pictures come into your mind. Any shape, any texture, any movement? If there is a shape or texture or movement, simply observe it. It may change. It may express something.

Is there a colour or feeling? Notice if there is. Don't do anything: keep breathing in air and light, keep focusing your attention, and letting go of any attempts you make to 'do' something or 'find' something.

You may get a sense there is something your pain needs to help it heal: wetness, soothing, unknotting, heat, whatever. If you want to, try imagining the thing the pain needs and give it to the pain. (For example, to soothe it, try a gentle dose of imaginary syrup, or ointment.)

Take enough time, even if nothing seems to happen at all. Try not to judge anything. Return to normal awareness when ready.

You may find that even if 'nothing happened' you now feel good about contacting your pain—maybe even relieved that you managed it without any scars to show for your efforts. Perhaps you found yourself going all over the place as you followed the pain. Perhaps you felt suddenly in touch with some strong emotions—and you are still feeling affected by them. Don't forget to share your feelings if you need to. If you can't share them with another—write them down and share them with yourself.

Trust that what you have done and what you have learned is of value.

Listening and Accepting

The strongest healing force in the world is love. Learning to accept and love ourselves, in all our mess and pain is really what illness is about. Letting ourselves look at the raw bones of ourselves and feel: Yes, this is *me*. If we discover we are a rather tatty old Ford not a Rolls Royce—this is the 'us' we need to love. If when we explore our voices, our feelings, we find they are ugly and difficult—this is the 'us' we need to love.

In the same way, if as soon as we start to look inwards at our centres, or our pain, we find ourselves feeling restless, irritated, bored, anxious or scared—this is the 'us' we need to love. These feelings—these expressions of ourselves—are worth staying with. There's no use in rushing off to hear some wonderful wisdom from some 'hidden' part of ourselves, meanwhile ignoring (not listening to, not hearing) the first words we speak.

Similarly we are merely repeating a pattern if we start off determined to prove that we have no centre, no inner wisdom, and march right past our feelings of fear or anxiety. Begin where you are: every journey is exciting and the best ones are those we take for ourselves.

If you find yourself feeling anxious—listen to, love that anxiety. Poor old anxiety has something to say. Where is it? Is it the worrier in your head? Is it a tightening knot in your stomach? Is it a hurting in your heart? Is it a little child in your belly, clinging to her mother and staring at you with worried eyes? There is no need to go past the anxiety at all. Everything you need to know is in that anxiety. Stay with it, and love it—or rather love *you* for feeling it.

All these pictures I conjure up, all, these ways of looking at myself, contain my one and only wish: that you can love or accept whatever starting point you find in yourself, and from that beginning, the rest will unfold.

There is no right journey, only your journey. There is no 'perfect' health, only your health. There is no ultimate authority you can ask who will tell you if you are doing the right thing (though your inner centre, your contact with the Divine may help)—this is why you might as well give up trying and worrying about whether you have got it right, and instead, laugh. Laugh as often as you can. And the best thing is: the more foolish you are, the more you have to laugh about!

19

Illness on a Spiritual Plane

A pond lily looks beautiful because beauty is in its nature.
It pays not attention to its reflection on the water.

Sickness can occur on all levels of being: body, mind, emotions, and spirit. Not everyone by any means needs to consider the spiritual plane in their lives, but for some people not to think about it is to deny a vital part of themselves, of their living energy.

It may be that for some time you have been interested in spiritual ideas. You may know, deep inside, that your love of people, or of nature is a deeply spiritual thing. But perhaps there is a part of you which has always been sceptical. Perhaps you have been offended by certain behaviour you attach to 'religious people'. Perhaps you feel Divine Love does not fit in with your philosophy of life. Or maybe you are already religious, but are suffering some real doubts and confusions which you do not know how to face.

If your illness is stuck, it may well be a sign that now is the time to look at the spiritual side of your life—to allow the inner part of you to reach out with trust, so that you can open to the true unfolding of your life's journey. This may sound rather grand written down, and yet it is very simple.

We can emphasise the fear, the worry, the accurate and biting criticisms: we can emphasise the pain, the suffering, the deep despondency; or we can simply quieten right down, and allow ourselves to contact the sacred source within us which is simply there, and part of everything else which is also simply there, and allow ourselves to surrender—if just for a brief moment—to the beauty and love we find there.

If we can allow this we can know—if just for a brief moment —that everything is OK. No matter how hellish or difficult the life which surrounds us appears, inside everything is fine; just as it is, right now, deep inside us.

Imagine you are swimming in a river. You are swimming upstream and it is hard work, and you feel life is a struggle. Sometimes you go under and feel depressed. Sometimes you get angry because you can't get anywhere. Suddenly you decide to stop struggling and let the river take you. You never did this before because you felt that surrender was a defeat, it meant accepting things you could not accept, being walked all over, or losing out. But suddenly you decide that the direction of the river is not the same thing as the whirls and eddies on its surface, and you trust it. As you are moved along you discover that the journey takes you in a better direction than you could have ever imagined. Further, because you are no longer struggling you have much more time and energy to enjoy the journey. And finally, the feeling of being able at last to trust that the *universe cares for you* (just as it cares for every living thing) is more warm and delicious than you ever dreamed.

I am not telling you a theory—or trying to persuade you to follow a certain way of thinking; if you treat my words this way they may have no meaning. I am simply saying there is an experience which you could have simply by quietening right down which will expand your life and allow you to feel loved. The Love is so kind and beautiful it makes me want to laugh and cry all at once. And this love (which you may choose to call God) is so awesome and sacred it fills you right up.

Whenever I am lost, whenever my life starts to fall apart, I realise sooner or later that I have forgotten to be close to this love. And as I go again through the process of opening, I find once more I have to go through my doubts, my scepticism, my anger at life. I find I have to keep letting go and letting go of the tension within me which resists opening out to the Divine. And it is my tension, my 'screwed-up-ness' which literally cuts me off from the ever present flow. Getting through this is not pleasant, and sometimes I give up in despondency and doubt. Luckily for me, something always brings me back—one moment and I'm through. And sometimes that 'something' has to be sharp enough to break through to me, and if I have become too 'asleep' the only thing which can pierce through me to my core, is suffering.

So there we are: suffering has become a tool which reminds me—no, which *helps* me to open to the one thing which can delight my entire being. Pain has become a stimulus which helps me persist in the developing and growing I must do to move closer to the Source.

A healer once said to me: "At least your pain reminds you you are alive." I could have murdered him at the time he said it, but his words stay with me, years later. I could add: 'At least your pain makes you desperate'. For when you are desperate you don't mess around; all the gloss, all the surface is gone, and you just have to go for the thing you need. You will even be prepared to take that step beyond, into the unknown, into the possibility that your mind, or your ego resists.

Our minds have worked hard all our lives to understand our surroundings, in order to be able to determine, to predict, to control. It is very hard for us to trust, literally to throw ourselves into the hands of the Divine, and then to appreciate the way our life turns out, appreciate what we are offered.

In reply to a questioner at one of his talks:"I'm afraid I may lose control,": Ram Dass replied "Let's hope so. I mean, which life do you want? Do you want an adventure, or would you like to make sure it comes out the way you thought it would?"

But if we are desperate enough, and we allow ourselves that moment of surrender, and the Love floods in, suddenly there is a whole new meaning to life, a new fullness to life, and we know how love really feels.

MAY WE BE OPEN

May we be open to the power of the Earth, the power that sustains our being.

May we be open to the light of the Universal Mind, the
power of creation.
May these great powers meet in us, and flow through us,
So that we may love Life and love the Earth more and more.
And through this love may rid the world of the selfishness,
which separates us from the rest of life.

(Paul Hawkins)

Whether the love comes from a Higher Intelligence, a God, or
from a kind of flame that burns within us, is merely an abstract
question. I have my own beliefs, but these are only to help me
stay close to the experience. And what counts for all of us is the
experience. What counts for me is that one evening I can be
feeling lonely and unloved, and then I open, and I feel good,
and full of love. One minute I can feel angry and bitter, and
then I experience the Love, and my hatred melts and is gone.

It is not about trying to be positive when you don't feel
positive at all, or 'looking on the bright side' if this means
ignoring very real horrible truths. It is about being exactly who
you are, where you are, and still feeling the Love coming to
you, without blame or judgement.

For there isn't any blame or guilt, but only the continual
remembering to open ourselves and be in touch with the
Source so that we can feel alive, can appreciate our lives, can
care about ourselves. From the experience of being loved, no
matter what state we are in, comes a natural desire to express
this love to other people, and to care about the very beautiful
world in which we find ourselves.

Giving ourselves permission to experience beauty in this
world is strangely, quite a difficult thing. Actually allowing
ourselves to spend time raising the level of beauty and love in
our environment is also a difficult thing. How many times do
we let our fears, worries, or criticisms intervene and 'bring
things down'?

In India they name talking together of the Divine, beauty
and love, 'Satsang'. In my little book I have included many
quotations which I feel give the 'texture', the 'taste', or
experience of Divine Love, in the hope that by reading them
you will feel 'uplifted', cheered in some deep way. In other

words I wish you to allow the words to touch you, soften you, and give you joy. In that state you are more able to get well. The more you can concentrate on this kind of beauty, the more you create a healing environment for yourself.

Sometimes we have lost the ability to pay attention to our spiritual side. We think we will meditate, but we watch television instead. We think we will make a lovely meal for our family; and we end up arguing with one of them and spoiling it, because we lose sight of the harmony we wanted. Something comes up at work, and we do it grudgingly, instead of saying no and giving ourselves what we really needed (or indeed, instead of doing it with a full heart). Then we have to literally *develop the habit* of paying our spiritual side attention. We actually have to *spend time* reading uplifting things, being quiet within ourselves, creating beauty which makes us feel good. Even in difficult circumstances we can give ourselves moments of beauty, if we choose consciously where we put our attention.

If you feel you are ill on the spiritual level, it may be you need to do something quite practical: increase the amount of time you spend with your attention in this area. During my last illness I discovered that the only thing that kept me from falling apart, kept me moving in a steady way towards health, was praying and meditating. Not thinking about it, not reading about it, even, but doing it. And believe me, I began doing it only because I wanted to get well, not because I had any faith. My spirituality up to then had been ideas, ideals, not practice. Once again, I owe it to my illness that I actually began to spend time doing something which nowadays is integral to my life. If the time is right for you, these words will touch you.

> Dislodging a green nut from a shell is almost impossible, but let it dry and the lightest tap will do it.
>
> (Ramakrishna)

Often in life we have a dream, and we set about achieving it. Perhaps it is having a house of our own, perhaps it is achieving in our work, perhaps it is having a 'good time'. At first putting our energy into this dream brings out the best in us. But it can happen that gradually the impulses that made us so awake, so vital, so creative, come to be drowned in the actual material thing we create. For example—the house which is decorated the way we wanted, filled with the furniture we worked so hard to get, which once was a source of 'safety' and joy to us, may become a responsibility which seems to encourage us to worry and feel anxious in case we should not be able to meet it.

Without the spiritual side to life, the way to conventional happiness is by doing more things, or collecting more things (or people). Yet we know that at any time these things could disappear, so this way fills us with fear, unrest, knowing we can't actually rely on any of the things we are building up. And because of this fear, instead of being able to simply enjoy these possessions, we spend a large amount of time counting them, guarding them, even working out ways to keep them safe from other people.

In our hearts we may be generous, we may care about others, but as soon as we are surrounded by things, we are in a position where we want to keep them separate from others, so they can be ours. Thus it is that in a country so full of material wealth, people are still suffering from lack:

> There is hunger for ordinary bread, and there is hunger for love, for kindness, for thoughtfulness; and this is the great poverty that makes people suffer so much.
>
> (Mother Teresa: *A Gift For God*)

Once we open to the spiritual side of life things, or the lack of them, seems to fall into their right perspective. We have more than we know, already. Financial gain is not a sure sign of success as a person. In fact it is harder to be loving when you are surrounded by possessions. When we have nothing we have to give of ourselves: time, love, care, because we have no things to offer. This is of course, why many spiritual disciplines call for giving everything up to dedicate one life to God, or Buddha and so on.

> One of Junaid's followers came to him and offered him a purse containing five hundred gold pieces.
> "Have you any more money than this?"asked the Sufi.

"Yes, I have."

"Do you desire more?"

"Yes, I do."

"Then you must keep it, for you are more in need than I; for I have nothing and desire nothing. You have a great deal and still want more."

(Idries Shah: *The Way of the Sufi*.)

In our own lives we sort out the balance as best as we can. But once we take the spiritual aspects of our lives into account we need to ask: do I own my possessions, or do they own me? Do they help me be more myself, or do they take me away from myself? Do they help me be more able to love, or make me less able to love? I know of one man who at 75, sold or gave away everything he owned and went travelling. I know a woman who by finding her inner calm was able to provide the material things she and her family longed for. The truth about your needs resides in your heart, if you listen. Opening to the spiritual plane for you may well mean resolving some inner conflict about your direction in life: and with the calm which follows, the calm in the knowledge of your closeness with the Divine path of your life, your healing can take place.

And he (Jesus) said unto her, Daughter be of good comfort; thy faith hath made thee whole; go in peace.

(Luke 8: 48).

Notice that Jesus did not say: "God hath made thee whole" or "I have made thee whole" but "*thy faith* hath made thee whole." It is your act, your willingness to open and surrender, which will open the way for your spirit.

20

Using Your Will

A great deal of chaos in the world occurs because people don't appreciate themselves. Having never developed sympathy or gentleness towards themselves, they cannot experience harmony or peace, and therefore, what they project to others is also inharmonious and confused. Instead of appreciating our lives, we often take our existence for granted or we find it depressing or burdensome. People threaten to commit suicide because they aren't getting what they think they deserve out of life...certainly we should take our lives seriously, but that doesn't mean driving ourselves to the brink of disaster by complaining about our problems, or holding a grudge against the world—we have to accept personal responsibility for uplifting our lives.

(Chogyam Trungpa)

Imagine for a moment that you accept responsibility for everything that happens to you today. What does this mean? Suppose a friend said they would call and they don't—is that your responsibility? Or is it simply your responsibility how you react to the circumstances? If you pretend you didn't mind when you did, is that your responsibility? If you are angry and they feel hurt then is that your responsibility?

Being responsible for your own life means the opposite of taking the weight of the world on your shoulders. Being responsible for our own lives does not mean blaming ourselves

142

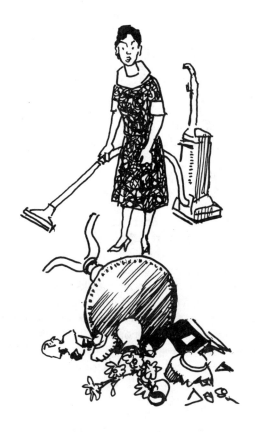

for anything that goes wrong in our lives, but nor does it mean blaming others. Blame does not come into it.

Taking responsibility simply means: no longer looking around for reasons why our life is as it is, but simply accepting it *is as it is*, and also accepting *we have the inner power to change it if we want to*. Not by struggling against things we don't like, or know are wrong, with the attitude that if *they change* everything will be all right—but instead by coming to know and love ourselves.

We cannot make a journey to Paris unless we know where we are journeying from. If we think we are in New York when we really are in London, we will never get where we want to be.

Are we really so anxious not to be in charge of our lives? Or is it because we avoid getting to know ourselves, we can't know what effect we have on the world, and therefore we can't really be responsible.

It's a bit like driving a car and not knowing when we push the accelerator whether it's top speed is 10 or 90 miles an hour. So we aim for the end of the road and press down, and get there without being sure just why people shake their fists at us on the way—or conversely just why they loved us. If we know a little of how the car works, and how to make it go fast or slow, we stand a much better chance of making the journey we intended to make. Furthermore when we drive we can then choose whether we drive carefully and safely or recklessly and dangerously. If we choose the latter, we can't turn round and blame others if we have an accident.

A Metis Medical Society teaching talks about being at the *cause* of life, not the *effect*. By this is meant being the one who initiated the events we experience, rather than being the one who experiences events other people initiated.

Of course it is not possible to just decide to be like this and—hey presto—no problems! Deciding you are going to change your attitude to yourself is hard; it takes discipline, and patience.

It takes the ability to stand back and watch yourself. It takes the willingness to open your heart and feel the pain within you. It take the willingness to love yourself for all the human parts of yourself, not just for the special or clever bits.

It takes a desire to experience the fullness of life. It takes a willingness to accept limitation and change, perhaps both at once. Far from being some lofty distant ideals, it is possible for you right now to make the commitment to grow closer to yourself, closer to life.

None of these things are special. They are all simple. They begin with an appreciation of life as something sacred and wonderful; as the most precious gift offering unlimited potential. Flowers which bloom in so many dazzling colours, filling the sweet air with delicate and strange perfume. Trees which create such lyrical harmony. Animals with soft eyes and loving touch, animals whose wild vigour makes your spirit lift and dance. The dark warmth of the earth, sparkling water—all this on this beautiful planet. So if you can't always appreciate the smile on a child's face, the closeness of friends and loved ones—there is so much more besides!

Opening our hearts and allowing ourselves to be touched by the world around us is the only way to understand its beauty. But remaining aware, and open, is not an act of bleary surrender, it is an act of discipline, of will. There is so much in this world to lull us to sleep. Pressures which knock us off centre. Confusion, dishonesty, fear which trip us up and make us lose the true needs of our spirit. Staying in touch with the honest truth about yourself takes determination. Not struggle, not tension, but a strong inner desire. The strength of this desire comes out from our thoughts, but from the area in our body where our will resides: our hara, our belly. When our mind is skidding about afraid and defeated, we need only to contact our pelvic area to find our inner strength. This strength does not come from us, so much as from our connection with life. What is good for life is good for us. To this end we may choose to say: 'I want, but life knows best.' or 'Whatever God will, will be done.'

> We must remember we are not intended to rely entirely on our own power, but rather to ask what constitutes right action. Ask through prayer, through addressing your own knowing, the Witness self, the Watcher within. Once you are clear, you can *neutralise your refusal to let right action flow through you*. Not intent on movement, be content to wait; while you wait, keep on removing resistances. As the obstructions give way, all remorse arising from 'trying to make it happen' disappears.
>
> (Ralph Blum: *The Book of Runes*.)

This does not mean giving in and accepting Fate—it may sound like it because the phrase 'accepting fate' incorporates the idea that fate is bad, harmful, oppressive. And so it is if we use the idea of Fate to justify our own defeatism.

But vital to the idea of aligning our will to the Divine is the understanding that we have power, and must be careful to use it to help the sacred balance of life, not go against it, and by so doing, only the best can happen.

The best may not always be the easiest or the nicest. What we need may not always be what we want. For example, though you are having to suffer illness, this is the best opportunity for you to come to know and love yourself. Suffering may force us to open our hearts and learn to give love in a way we never could have managed before. Countless people achieve wonderful things *because* of something terrible which has happened to them.

Please do not think I am saying this lightly. I know there is great suffering involved, and I would not wish suffering on anyone. I do not understand why we have to have pain—or at least so much pain—on this life's journey.

I *can* begin to see that I create a lot of the pain I experience in life for myself. I can also see that other people do this too—and I can increase my own pain if I expect people to be any better at living than I am—because I am only setting myself up for disappointment. But I also experience the truth that the more I love myself, the more I love life, the more I surrender to the unfolding of the Divine, the better life becomes.

Perhaps one of the pleasures of being ill is that once you start to recover, you really appreciate your new found health. Suddenly your being out of pain becomes a precious gem you really value.

You realise that being able to get out of bed and walk around is a gift. Many people never walk. And if you can't walk, you know that being able to move around again is a gift; to move from one scene to another; to look out of a window; to breathe in fresh air. What gifts!

> There are so many people who can come up with an idea of how we 'ought to be', or the 'ideal society', or the 'ideal human being'. And there are plenty of people who can go out there and say, "By the way guys, this is how we ought to be." No shortage of it. And all I do is I carry a little mirror with me, and anytime somebody says "Well, how should I be?

What should my goals be?" I just try to whip out that little mirror and say: "Look do you even know what you have?" And then people can take a simple look at a very simple life, at a very simple concept of being alive, of being here—it's very, very simple, it is so simple, so sweet, and so kind. Because it's only human beings who can take a coconut and say "I wonder what the purpose of a coconut is?" While everybody else on the beach might be enjoying themselves by drinking the milk from the coconut, enjoying the middle part, there are some people who are starving and at the same time wondering what the purpose of a coconut could possibly be. If a coconut falls on one of their heads, that person writes down "The purpose of a coconut is to hit you on the head." If one falls on the foot, somebody says, "No, no, no no. We're all mistaken. The purpose of the coconut is to fall on the foot, not on the head." And then somebody gets hit on the shoulder and says, "The ideal use of the coconut is to throw it at your enemies when they're coming too close." But all they have to realise is that all along, all through this, the purpose is that enjoyment that life is offering, every single day.

Being able to be thankful is such an art. By the way guys, it's not so easy as we think. It really isn't, "Gee whiz, just go out there and be thankful." It really isn't. Life is immaculate and so has to be its appreciation. Immaculate.

(Maharaji. *Elan Vital newsletter.*)

21

Listening to Baby Self

The belly is a very sacred place. In the days when our forebears used to worship the Goddess, she was often depicted with a huge belly. What we as a people admired was her ability to create life—was her fertile, powerful centre.

The belly is not only a source of life, but also—for each of us—a source of energy. It is as if we have a flame ever burning at the base of our spine, which dies to a tiny flicker when we are ill—and when we are well, flares up beautiful, passionate, creative and golden.

Too often we allow our active, mental preoccupations—particularly self-criticism and worry, to drain the energy from this flame, so that we feel sapped, depressed, lifeless.

When we are ill we often take the time to read books, or watch TV, in part for enjoyment, and in part to take our minds away from our pain. This is fine—it's great—but we need to be careful not to stay in our thoughts all day long, ending up feeling headachey, dull and tired.

If our belly is empty of joy, of desire—we need to spend some time replenishing ourselves. Meditation will; so will making beautiful things—sewing, drawing etc. Even having a bath, smelling flowers, smiling, laughing, all these activities will help our bellies fill-up.

Consciously thinking of our belly area filling with energy is another way. If you try this you may notice how little attention this part of you normally receives. Imagine the flame at the base of your spine—and imagine it flaring up and glowing, in

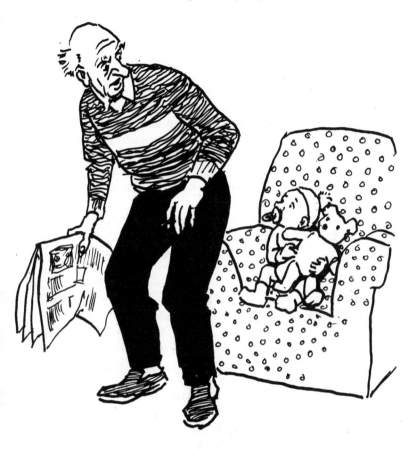

the air and water of your pelvis, until the area is beautiful and bright.

When we made our Goddesses of old we were no doubt expressing our worship of women's real ability to grow life and give birth, but it is my belief that all of us have, within our own belly, within our own energy centre, a kind of personal baby: we are all of us pregnant with the baby part of ourselves.

Many years ago I spent the evening with two women friends, telling them of my longing to have another child, and expressing my sadness because the time wasn't right. My longing then was so fierce, it literally used to hurt me. It was like a desperate need, a hunger which I was always searching to satisfy. I felt it was a very basic female instinct, and was very angry at being thwarted by life—and very sorry for myself.

We began to talk about why I was so desperate. No one denied it was a wonderful thing to have a baby. No one thought my desire strange. But, we wondered, why the desperation? We talked about the way we all longed to give our love and attention to someone little who needed us. Then we began to explore the idea that we too wanted that love and attention. Perhaps inside us was a baby aspect of ourselves to which we could give the love and attention we were wanting to give to a real baby?

Many women seem to give so much love to their children, and so little to themselves. When my son was young I sometimes used to give him his tea, and then assume I had fed myself.

Many people—men and women—continue to deny the baby part of themselves attention, imagining they must be 'grown up' now and not have needs and wants. Meanwhile their baby-self keeps sneaking out and asking other people for attention. (Maybe this is why some wives of seemingly big strong men can be heard to say 'He's just a big baby'.)

Giving our own baby-self attention is *not* the same as giving our ego attention, it is not the same as being egotistic and self-centred. In fact it's almost the opposite: many egotistic people appear to be like spoilt if charming children, they have never learned to grow up and give their baby-self attention, so they go round expecting and demanding it from everybody else.

Part of growing up is learning to stop looking to other people to fulfil all our needs and to start finding ways to care for ourselves. (This doesn't mean we don't want other people's love—or company). Finding our baby-self is a great help in this journey because we can't meet our own needs until we meet all the parts of us that are needful, and our littlest self is often pretty needy.

But why do we have to meet our own needs? Why can't we just meet the 'right person' who'll satisfy all our needs? The point is that when we were babies we needed love, harmony, understanding and attention from our parents or carers. It may be—for many reasons—you did not get the love or attention you needed. Maybe you were loved, but not understood. Maybe you were loved, but not enough. Maybe you did not feel loved.

Whatever the situation, by the time you were five or six years old, the inner pattern of your nature, your self, was pretty much set—after that time, no matter how much someone else wants to, *no one can turn back the clock and give you what you missed as a child.*

If they try, they will never seem to do it right, they will never seem to understand (as if they could understand, just like a parent, without your telling them). The point is: they can't: the only person who can understand and do it right is *you.*

You alone can give your baby what it needs. And if you do, that part of you will become less needy, and grow into the fine human being it is meant to be. I can find my baby-self when I take my attention down into my belly. She is an expression of my basic instincts. I give her a being and a character because it helps me to visualise which bit of me I'm dealing with. I call her 'baby-self' because she behaves just like a child: with tactless honesty. She is the part of me likely to say 'I'm fed up, I want to go home' in the middle of a friend's party, while I go round smiling politely at people I hardly know. She is part of me that yells 'No, no, no' and wants to kick her feet and have a tantrum, while I labour away in my grown up voice to explain why I disagree with my partner. She is the part of me that brightens up my day by whisking me into the shop to buy those glittering earings or bar of chocolate or whatever.

While the rest of our being is often easily persuaded by our head's logic, she never is. But unfortunately she's so little that we often ignore her. If we learn to listen, though, we are guaranteed to find out what our basic untempered feelings are. We might not like them, and we may want to modify them, but we'll probably be shocked at their accuracy.

And finally, if we learn to listen to her, we'll no longer find she sneaks out at just the wrong moment, and sabotages all the nice order our brain has just set up. And we might just enjoy her sense of fun too!

22

Despair

To find joy is not to banish despair; unless you are highly developed, like Mother Teresa, who is so busy loving she has no time for despair.

For most of us, during a long illness, there will inevitably be those grey, grey days, when all that we have begun to feel good about vanishes in a puff of smoke one early morning when we wake up to find we are worse, not better.

Despair is like a damp chill creeping through our bones. In moments of despair we can't even do the things for ourselves—such as call a friend, pray, meditate—which would make us feel better. That is the power of despair—it takes away our faith in life.

When you wake in despair—and if you are ill you are lucky if you never do—don't be afraid to sink further into it. Sometimes all we can do is allow it to wash over us like polluted sea, and wallow in it. Wallow in our own hopelessness.

If you allow yourselves to fall as far as you can you will hit the bottom. From there the only way is up. In your despair, you may find your baby-self is the part of you which helps you most. Though she will probably be the loudest winging voice of all, she may also provide you with a way of helping yourself.

Perhaps she'll want a sweater, or something else to cuddle. Perhaps she'll demand chocolates or something else she knows you don't approve of. Perhaps she'll want to go under the bedclothes and hide. Perhaps she wants to suck her thumb. When I was ill and in pain I took to sucking my thumb sometimes when I needed comfort. I also took to clutching a quartz crystal. Sometimes all we can do is hang on. Just let the moments pass us by, stroke our hair, listen to the clock, and wait.

It is said that suffering gives us more compassion for others. It is known amongst healers that we are often best at healing those things we've experienced ourselves.

You can't always avoid the dark blue days of depression. But if you can let yourself lie there clutching your pillow, maybe snivelling like a little hurt baby, maybe just staring, you will find something very deep happen inside you—some inner sense that it is even OK to be depressed, because most of all, it's OK to be human.

EMERGING

At the bottom
in the raw
stay still and time will pass
watch and listen
Nothing more

The centre has a long way to come
emerging
something is coming
emerging
Just watch and listen
Stay still and wait for the day
it splashes up

No idea
how much more
what to expect
holding on to nothing
at the bottom
in the raw.

23

Getting Well

Getting well again is a peculiar process. We are no sooner free of some of the pain or discomfort than we've forgotten what it was like. It's strange how our memory can't retain the experience of pain—it's only if it comes back again that we say: 'Oh, no, I'd forgotten how horrible this was!'

And yet for a long time into the journey of getting well *we still feel ill*. We are aware of the symptoms which have not improved, not the ones which have. Particularly if we have been ill for any length of time, coming back into the world feels like a delicate and difficult process.

For a start, if we've spent a long time lying down, our muscles will have weakened, and our sense of balance grown accustomed to being horizontal not vertical. We can't put back the muscle tone we've lost, overnight. We have to take care of ourselves—guard the gains we've made, try to make sure we don't overdo it and slip backwards.

We may feel particularly vulnerable to groups of people. We've been more or less alone for a long time, and being amongst people again may throw us temporarily off balance. It is very interesting to note just *how much* of an effect other people have on you. This is going on when you are well, too, but maybe you don't usually notice.

Use your extra sensitivity to work out which people you find most stimulating, which people you find most draining. Do

154

you find stimulating people also make you feel safe, or not? What kind of things do you feel are demanded of you by other people? Do you feel the need to entertain them? To take on their burdens and sort out their problems? To protect them? To impress them? Notice whether you are moving away from your centre when you talk to them. Do you lose a sense of who you are, or gain one? Do all your resolves go out the window, or do other people help you keep to them? Are you able to feel happy and centred at the same time? Does excitement help or hinder your recovery?

This is a good time for you to practise making your limitations clear. This is the time to see if you can say 'no' without sounding (or feeling) either apologetic, resentful or angry. (This is very difficult. There is a course called assertiveness training, which is designed precisely to help you over this issue, and if you discover that you find this very difficult when you 'experiment' now, you may like to find out more about it.)

It is important not to be angry at other people for not knowing how ill or well you are. They do not know what you can manage—no one knows but you. And you may not be very good at knowing that either! When we are recovering we are still 'raw' and 'vulnerable' from all those days in bed, and giving ourselves extra protection and attention is *only right and sensible*.

Sometimes people may say the most distressing things in an attempt to 'buck you up' or encourage you to be well. Things which end up making you feel a failure ('I should be better; he says he was at my stage') or angry ('How does she know what my illness feels like!) or sad ('I wish I was well, no one likes me when I'm weak and useless'.)

Sometimes it is difficult to remember that other people feel vulnerable too. Some people can't cope with illness—it brings out all their fears of ever being in your position, and they hurriedly try to prove to you by their words or behaviour that they won't be. Some people feel inadequate—they don't know how to express their caring. Or even at times they are (albeit unconsciously) jealous of the attention you are giving yourself, because they would really like to give themselves the same. (These are often the very people who talk about ill people being self-indulgent, or say they 'don't have the time to be ill'!)

No matter. Let it go again. You are at this stage in your life—they will be very lucky if they avoid going through it themselves at some time, but they may not have got there yet. You, on the other hand, have now developed an inner compassion, which means you *will* react to someone else when they are ill in future.

So, let it go. Let their words float away. You are the important person at the moment. If it helps you, try imagining you are surrounded by a beautiful ring of light which encircles and encloses you from head to foot, so that anything they direct at you simply deflects off the light, and leaves you untouched.

Remember that most advice is someone's opinion formed from his experience of himself and life. Before you listen to his advice, decide whether his approach *suits you*, and whether you think this person *cares for himself* in a way you would like to care for yourself. If he doesn't care for himself he will find it hard to care for you—even if he means to—because his fears and projections will get in the way.

If something anyone says hurts you, the important thing is for you to *to rescue the bit of you that is hurting, and not to use their words to go on and on upsetting yourself.* This is true even if you end up thinking what he said was right.

There are a lot of steps you can take to help yourself keep on getting well, once you have started. In some ways, beginning to recover is the most testing part of the whole illness. Because the pain or sickness is not so severe we no longer have a heavy hand restraining our every move. Our old habits and ways of approaching life seem to be jostling with each other, waiting to jump in and take over the show. Once more we find ourselves starting to plan for the future. All the things we've put aside seem to be asking for attention.

It isn't simply people you have to protect yourselves from either, but all the complexities of modern life. Going out of your house, walking down the road, you may hardly feel strong enough to deal with crossing the road, let alone buying your groceries. It is difficult to believe how much energy everything seems to take. How tiring standing in a queue can be!

Recovery has always been the hardest part of an illness for me, and it has taken me many years to learn the basic rules I'm about to share with you. There is no doubt a lot more I still don't know about.

Stop Before you are Full

Better to stop short than fill to the brim
Oversharpen the blade, and the edge will soon blunt:
Amass a store of gold and jade, and no one can protect it.
Claim wealth and titles and disaster will follow.
Retire when the work is done.
This is the way of heaven.

(Lao Tsu *Tao Te Ching.*)

The American Indians describe everything in the Universe in terms of circles. An easy circle to think of is the seasons: Spring, Summer, Autumn, Winter, Spring... If we put the seasons on a clock face, or circle, we can (just for the sake of this example) start at the bottom for winter, and work our way round clockwise to the top, for summer:

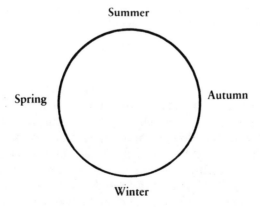

Summer

Spring   Autumn

Winter

As we move from the bottom, we move into spring, with the weather hopefully getting gradually warmer, until we reach twelve o'clock, the height of summer. The next thing that happens, if we go any further round the circle, is that we start to move back down again, on our way into autumn, then winter. This is true of all energy: It rises, comes to a peak, and subsides. The thing is to notice that at its height (12 o'clock) is exactly when it is actually *beginning to subside*.

Now many people quite naturally understand this about their own energy. They instinctively stop before they begin to lose out. My son, who is extremely healthy, is like this. He is the only child I know who can go into a penny arcade and come out with more pennies that he went in with!

But some of us do not find it easy to know when to stop. Our instinctive reaction is to go on and on until we drop—and only after we are too tired do we realise we have overdone it yet again! For those of you who—like me—need to be told, this is the secret: stop before you are full. Withdraw while the going is good. Oversharpen the blade and it will soon blunt!

One of the problems is that it is *enjoyable* to find that we suddenly have energy. Especially if we have been ill for a long time, it is exciting to find we can do the things we've been deprived of: we rush around—like the child balancing on her bicycle who has suddenly found she can use 'no hands', grinning excitedly, telling everyone: "Look at me, I can do it!" The only thing is, though, you know what happens to the child on the bike if she gets too over-excited—yes, of course,—she crashes into something, or overbalances and falls off. It's in the nature of things, I'm afraid.

So the trick is: as soon as you feel self-confident and good, catch yourself and stop. This does not mean: keep undermining yourself *at all*. If you go on at this point, *that is when you undermine yourself* because you start to waste all you have gained. Enough is enough. And learning to 'catch' that moment when to do any more would be too much, is an incredible skill, and an extremely difficult one to achieve too. If going 'over the circle' is your tendency, don't expect you can change it overnight. It takes a good deal of vigilance to begin to notice the point where you have moved from 11.30 to 12.00

o'clock. It has something to do with accepting endings. As a child my mother says I never wanted anything to finish. As an adult I still find it hard to 'leave when the work is done', to let something go on without me.

But to say 'no more now', and retire from the stage does not mean missing out. A more efficient use of energy gives you more to use in the long run. Again, the important point about stopping is: stopping with love. Too often 'no' is connected in our minds with being limited or deprived, instead of being helped and loved. To say no is to remember our main purpose—and this is to maintain enough energy to say yes when we need to.

Save energy for your Health

Doing some things gives you more energy than others, and this doesn't have to have anything to do with the muscle power it takes. (Similarly being with some people gives you more energy than being with others.) If you find that doing something gives you a boost of energy—once again: *stop*, don't go rushing off madly and spending it!

Imagine you have the energy egg inside and you are two thirds full, perhaps three quarters full, because you are in the process of recovering. Something 'sets you on fire' making you feel happy and excited, and suddenly you don't feel ill at all—you feel you could walk to the moon and back!

Instead of setting off for the moon, and realising you weren't quite up to it half way there: STOP, and allow yourself to feel the excitement and energy boost rushing and bubbling about inside you. Contain that energy and imagine it flowing to all the parts of you which are still unwell, and healing them.

When people talk about life being a flow, and letting energy flow through you—they are describing what can happen when you have a full energy egg inside you. But when your body needs repairing, your first job is to give all your energy excess to YOU. Of course in the Universe this still leaves extra energy around, because if you put that energy into making yourself better, someone else won't have to, and that leaves them free to give it to someone else.

Keep an eye on your Worry Patrol

Sometimes healers talk about energy 'leaking out' of people. You could visualise that as your energy egg with lots of tiny holes in it. One of the ways you can leak energy out of yourselves—energy which could be helping you recover—is by worrying. Of course you may have lots of things that seem to justify worrying about and I am not suggesting you try to ignore them and walk about with a false smile on your face.

Worries are worries. But unless the worry is an emergency, we are often unable to do anything about it immediately. In fact you could almost say that is the essence of a worry: it is something *you can't* (or won't) *do something about immediately*, so it keeps swishing round and round in your head. Sometimes it is better to go ahead and have a good old fullblown worry for ten minutes, and preferably share it with someone—than to try to ignore it.

If you watch your brain working, you may be amazed to find how often worry patrol marches up and down, parading your worries, and how clever it is: because once one has been dealt with, there is always another one to take its place.

As often as you can, notice when you are worrying and decide to let it go. This is not the same as trying to ignore it, or push it away. It is a far more comforting feeling. It's more of a 'That worry again, Tessa, give yourself a break'. You notice that—once again—the extra quality is love. Out of concern for ourselves, we put our worries to one side. Or: out of concern for ourselves we first do what we can to solve our worries (and this may be nothing at all if we don't feel well) and then we put them to one side. Just realising that worries are an energy drain may help you to resist dwelling on them all the time.

Even if it is a pressing worry *it is ok not to worry about it all the time*. There is nothing feckless or careless about giving yourself a space away from your worries. In fact it is that space which will actually help you deal with them. Sometimes we develop a habit of always having something to worry about. When you were ill maybe you didn't have enough spare energy to keep this habit up all the time (or maybe worrying about dying drove all the other worries out of the competition), but now you are better you have settled into it without noticing.

What would you do without worries to worry about? Would you feel safe? Sometimes worrying feels like our little bargain with the world: 'I promise to go on worrying about all the small things, and if I do, World, promise not to spring anything too big on me.' If you stop worrying for a moment, your world will not end. You can still breathe. Still look around you. So, you owe the bank manager money—but you are still you, still able to look up and see your favourite picture, or see that child laughing, or the colour of those flowers.

You can't stop worrying by worrying about it, that is why you have to 'put it aside'. And if you are a great worrier, maybe you could let someone else help you. Instead of putting it aside—hand it over to the Lord, to Christ, to your Bhudda nature, to the Universe. Hand it over, and be comforted.

> Yes, though I walk through the valley of the shadow of death, I will fear no evil: for thou art with me; thy rod and thy staff they comfort me.
>
> (Psalm 23)

Allow Things to 'Do' Themselves

Practise non action
Work without doing
Taste the tasteless
Magnify the small, increase the few
Reward bitterness with care.

See simplicity in the complicated.
Achieve greatness in little things.
In the Universe the difficult things are done as if they are easy
In the Universe great acts are made up of small deeds.
The sage does not achieve anything very big, and thus achieves greatness.

Easy promises make for little trust
Taking things lightly results in great difficulties,
Because the sage always confronts difficulties
He never experiences them.

(Lao Tsu: *Tao Te Ching*)

How do we work without doing? Most people when they set about a task, put in many times more effort than they need to. Effort in terms of hundreds of tense muscles, effort in terms of over-concentrating on getting to the end (thus producing anxiety, aggravation, even panic) instead of enjoying the journey.

My Alexander Technique colleague would argue that this is a historic body pattern: that is, once we have started to use our body with excessive tension, this becomes a habitual body pattern, which in turn leads to using ourselves with tension, and so forth. Without lessons in the technique, which help you physically experience using your body with less effort and tension, a person can't 'throw off' their old pattern of use just because they want to, or because they think it is a good idea.

Certainly the Alexander Technique is perhaps unique in that it can give you the experience of 'work without doing', and teaches you how to follow that experience yourself. And it may be true that for some people there is no way to move past years of tension, just by wanting to, or understanding the need to. I say this because I don't want you to feel a failure if you can't easily get the hang of 'work without doing'. I certainly didn't. However, the sages were putting this idea forwards long before the Alexander Technique was developed, and they obviously hoped the saying of it (so beautifully) would help you achieve it, and I do too.

Work without doing. Allow things to do themselves. Work without doing. Let the motion of the thing you have begun carry itself forward of its own volition. You don't have to stand over a kettle and shake it to get it to boil ('a watched kettle never boils'), you simply let it boil itself. You don't have to huff and puff and scrunch up your shoulders with tension in order to drive a car, you can allow the car to drive you along.

You don't have to worry and struggle to please a child, to control her, to look after her: you can allow the child to look after herself (with a little love and help from you), and allow her to entertain herself, or be entertained by things you are already doing, for yourself. And better still: allow yourself to be entertained by her. You don't have to check up every loose end and anticipate every disaster ten times over—if you stay with your centre you can let things go along their own sweet way, and only act when it is needed. Step by step, small step by small step. Life can be easy. Not expecting everything to go right, nothing can go wrong, only differently.

See how many times a day you can resist the temptation to interfere with something someone else is doing. See how many times a day you can trust that the thing you set in motion will be alright. The world has been rolling along for millions of years and it really can get on fine without us!

Listen, Don't Entertain

The ability to entertain people and make them laugh is a rich and wonderful gift. But when you are ill or recovering, you don't have to be the one who does the entertaining. Some people talk out of a deep inner habit. They feel anxious if there is a silence: they feel it is up to them to fill it. Sometimes they even feel they have to make the other person happy, to give them 'their money's worth'. Others encourage people to talk about their problems, and listen to them, out of a deep habit. They are trying to 'help' the other, trying to please the other by 'helping'.

The important word here is *habit*. We do these things not out of love, because it simply springs out of us; not out of the need of the moment, because it needs to be done, but out of habit, because we are trying to live up to some self-image we have of ourselves, without which we would feel lost and awkward. But habits are energy-drainers, because when we are in a habit, we are going along tramlines that feel so familiar we forget to look out and take notice. Afterwards we can feel almost as if something else took us over and acted for us.

Well, this is a good time to look at these habits, for they are keeping you from seeing something new about yourself or the world. (As all habits do.) Experiment a little. Imagine you are more ill than you feel yourself to be—create a little space—and imagine you can't do what you habitually would want to do. See what happens if you don't talk, or don't sympathise.

People react in various ways with different people. If, for

example, I visit someone who talks a lot, I tend to listen. If I visit someone who listens I tend to talk a lot. It is very exciting to discover that someone you thought you had to entertain, really has a lot of interesting things to say, and can entertain you. It is equally exciting to discover that someone who usually tells you all their problems, can move out of that and show you care, and talk about something else.

Also being with someone is not simply talking. We sometimes talk so much we don't communicate at all. Just sitting and being *with* someone, perhaps in silence, can be a very moving thing.

Keep Checking around your Body

You have hopefully by now learned to listen to at least some of the things that are going on in your body. Remember to listen to your heart centre to see how you are feeling. Notice the level of tension in your solar plexus. See whether you are in touch with your belly, your legs, your feet. Notice if your baby-self is happy. Perhaps you can visualise your body-egg; if so notice whether it is filling up or emptying.

You are not checking round your body as another way to worry about life, or as a way to become self-obsessed, or scared 'something will go wrong'. You are checking yourself like a monitoring system—making sure everything is running smoothly so that you can function well. If you learn to listen out, your body will learn that its messages are being heard, and will give them more readily.

Allow a Quiet Space

I need to give myself a quiet space away from my day, at least twice in a day, well or ill. That is, I need at some point to go to my room (or a church, or a field, or a park, or a beach) and either sit and just be myself, or sleep, or pray or meditate, or work on myself with the Alexander Technique.

There are so many stimulae in this world which cause stress and tension in our bodies. When we become involved in them we can easily become wound up and disconnected—that is we can easily lose a sense of contact with our inner selves and with the Divine Love which surrounds us, and start to struggle, or push, or grasp, or worry.

We can easily be knocked off balance by the fear and tension in other people (for example, our boss in a bad mood can upset our day). That is why having a quiet place to retreat to, even just for five or ten minutes, is so important.

It is only by taking yourself out of your environment and focussing all your attention on yourself that you can really know what is going on—especially when you are just beginning all this!

Although at first it may seem difficult to imagine giving yourself such spaces (only five minutes!), once you have started you may begin to enjoy them so much, you will miss them if you don't continue.

Keep an Overview

When you are ill, or recovering, you only have a limited amount of energy (money) in your bank account. Those of you who are good at staying in the black will appreciate that the only way to do this is: (a) to have a clear idea of just how much you have to pay out each week and (b) always to keep some extra for emergencies/surprises.

The same principles—exactly the same—apply to your health. It is no good spending all your energy today and leaving yourself weak and tired tomorrow.

Plan out your week—as much as you can—in advance. If Wednesday looks like a busy day, try to leave Tuesday and Thursday quiet. As much as possible, even out the load. Always be prepared to drop something if your energy level runs down. Remind yourself of your plans for the next day, today, so that you can finish this one well enough to get through tomorrow as well.

Be Flexible

The only thing you can't be flexible about right now is your health: YOUR HEALTH MUST COME FIRST. This means that everything else may or may not happen, depending on how you feel.

Try not to make too many fixed commitments. Try to leave yourself alternatives. Try not to become too attached to any one thing happening, because it is definitely sod's law that the one thing you are really attached to will be the one thing you have to give up!

This can be a very good teaching for us because we can learn that there are always alternatives to the plans in our heads. Change does not have to mean disaster. In fact it is a lovely thing to experience letting go of a plan and realising everything can still work out fine. What counts is not so much what happens, as our attitude towards it. It is a lovely thing to experience letting go of a plan, and seeing life unfold quite differently to the way we planned it, and to realise that the way it is unfolding is perhaps even better than our idea could have been.

We have to take care to make sure we *really* let go of plans once we see they are not feasible. If we spend all our time after we decide not to go to that meeting wondering what we are missing, and feeling cross and agitated about missing it—we might just as well have gone for all the good we've done ourselves!

If we relax, however, and let ourselves look at what we have left: there will always be something. Even the thought of a long evening's sleep can be enjoyable—if we see it that way, perhaps by making our bed extra nice and warm, changing our pillow case, or making ourselves a wonderful drink to take with us.

And any extra: well, meditation can be such an exciting experience. So can reading a book. It's a question of how willing we are to settle into the evening or day we do have, and leave the one we don't have behind.

It is a truly liberating experience to find yourself able to enjoy something which seemed to be a let-down. It helps you realise that it is our attachments and expectations in life which cause us more trouble than life itself!

Keep Loving Yourself

So you can't let go of your plans, you feel miserable or grumpy or both. OK. Fine, what can you salvage? Can you love yourself for it?

The most important part of getting well and staying well is to keep loving yourself. During the day when you check out your body, notice the way you are doing the checking—notice your attitude. We can do everything right, but if we do it for the wrong reasons, it won't turn out right anyway. The easiest way to sabotage anything is to swap an attitude of love for ourselves, for another attitude.

It is incredible how easy it is to do this! Suddenly we discover we are not acting out of love for ourselves, in order to be right; or to please or impress someone else; or because we feel we ought to; or because we feel we 'need improving' (aren't good enough); or because we don't like ourselves now...the list is endless, but the noticeable thing about all these attitudes is they all involve moving from the inner circle of our being, to the outer circles.

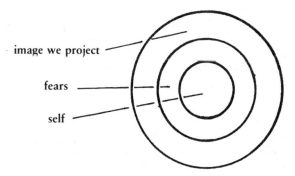

We have moved into thinking about how we appear to other people, how we compare with other people. Once we allow our life to be propelled by fears (of criticism, of someone not liking us if we don't please them) or by our self-image (that is what we should do, or an idea we want to project) we have lost our centre, and lost our loving attitude towards ourselves.

Without love towards ourselves, we are liable to do all sorts of things which will threaten our health again.

24

Invalid Consciousness

If, after being ill for a long time, and up and out of your bed for some time too, you still feel very shaky, it is worth considering whether you have developed a sort of invalid consciousness.

This may not apply to you, and it certainly is not a stick to beat yourself with. But sometimes if we have been ill and in pain for some time our body grows accustomed to being in a state of weakness and fearfulness. The last thing we want is a repeat dose of our pain or illness. So we limit our activity, and watch out for or avoid any situation which might threaten the stability we have managed.

Of course we need to feel better some of the time—without terrible pain or sickness—before we can go on to the next stage of being well. And it is far better to be over-cautious than push ourselves too hard and end up back in bed. But we can also develop an over-protectiveness, which means we don't stretch our body at all, and remain in a rather passive state. Sometimes this passivity can be self-perpetuating.

The answer is not to drop all caution and go for a four mile hike! What we need is a way of gently extending ourselves—gently increasing our physical activity and gradually all the limits we have around us. Gentle exercise in our rooms is a good place to start, so that we can flop down again if we are tired or worried about anything. Put on some music and make some gentle stretching movements. Dance a little. Enjoy the feeling. If you can get your heart-rate up a little, it is a good thing for it encourages more breath, a better circulation of the blood, and thus more energy. Sometimes a little burst of energy seems to break through the stagnation, and we feel a lot happier.

Remember, not to stretch muscles too much all at once, and do it consistently, every day. Remember that if this stretching and use leads to some slight aching, your body is probably only reacting normally, not going back to being ill again. Whatever you do, do it with love, enjoy it, and don't push yourself. Another activity is gentle walking, and also swimming: if you can get to a pool it is really worth overcoming the embarrassment and going in. Swimming is a lovely thing to do as well as being one of the best all-round exercises.

It is better, if you can, to try to build up the fitness of your body, before taking on your normal life—such as work. Fitness is an acquired thing for anyone, and can't be acquired without exercise. Don't forget that there are also healing therapies available, among them: yoga, massage, the Alexander Technique, which can help you gently encourage your body back to health.

Next, having encouraged you to listen to yourself and to your pain, I am now going to contradict myself (well, almost).

As you become well, it is important to spend time involved in something which takes your mind off your state of health, that helps you not to identify yourself as 'an ill person'. Find a place, or people who do not treat you as 'ill', where you can express other parts of your character apart from the fact that you suffer or are in pain. If you have been ill for a long time, perhaps a large amount of your life has become adapted to being ill, and so gradually even begins to reinforce your illness. What was a safe shelter, becomes a cocoon which begins to make you feel you can't go beyond it. It is alright to feel a little shaky as you step out on your first new experience for a while, its alright to feel a little nervous.

If you are able to avoid going straight back into a situation like work, or mothering, which feels too much all at once, perhaps you can arrange to do it by stages. If you are in a position to choose what you do—perhaps you could find somewhere where you could 'help out' for an hour or so—at a neighbour's, at the local school, or community centre, or club, or local church, somewhere where you can enjoy yourself and be of use, without feeling too over-responsible or too pressurized. Or again, just be with friends who do not notice your state of health, but who take your mind 'out of yourself' for some time.

After a deep journey inwards, we need to allow some time 'outwards' again. Not to the extent of throwing aside everything we have learned and gained, but simply to counteract any tendency for our world to become 'out of touch' and 'out of proportion'. As we recover we can begin to emphasise the parts of us which *can* function, don't hurt, can laugh, can be involved in life. In this way we begin to spread our interests beyond ourselves, and affirm one important fact: we are not simply who we are, we are also part of life itself, and we can participate—however briefly—in the world around us.

25

Setbacks

Though it is hard to believe when we experience it, getting first better then worse is all part of recovery. It is as if our body recovers by taking three steps forward, two steps back. In the same way that a child doesn't learn to walk except by falling down, we can't learn our limits and potential without going past them sometimes. So if you read this while you are lying in bed feeling miserable because you were well yesterday—the important thing to remember is: YOU WERE WELL YESTERDAY. That was a taste of things to come. Your body is telling you how well you can be—provided you allow yourself!

It may be that you have a clear idea of what it was you did yesterday (or the day before) which put too much strain on your system, and made you worse again. It doesn't necessarily need to be exercise that tires you out—sometimes it can give you energy. It may be that being with certain people tired you out—or that you returned to old habits of tension and worry and they made you tired. Perhaps you gave too much of yourself, trying to 'help' someone else. Or maybe you just don't know why: there have been plenty of times I haven't known why, and searching around for reasons just hasn't helped at all.

If you can, allow yourself to notice what it was, without getting too angry at yourself about it. Far better to say—"Oh, that's a good lesson, it teaches me something about what I do with my energy levels when I do..." (what ever it was), than to say: "you idiot, you've ruined everything!" Setbacks are almost inevitable—so don't be hard on yourself. See it as a time to shower yourself with love and sympathy. Groan and moan——but keep on knowing it is only a setback.

Your body is going in the direction of health, know that, and feel it in your heart. It may not be fast enough and constant enough for your liking but still, can you remember how ill you once were? You are getting there; really you are. Setbacks are only a pause, a lesser reminder of what you have left behind. Part of getting better is realising you can get ill again, and then recover *far quicker than before*.

Another aspect of getting better is: sometimes when the energy in our body is very low, our body saves all its resources to get through the basic day-to-day living. But as the energy level increases our body may decide to use some of the extra energy to tackle any left-over health problem. Thus the problem may seem to be getting worse, while it may simply be getting more attention.

Any of you who have been having Complementary Medicine treatments will know about the concept of healing crisis: the idea that things often have to get worse before they can get better. That often what we see as terrible symptoms: for example spots or catarrh are actually signs that our body is already in the process of making us well, by eliminating from our systems all the damaging poisons.

It might help to see your setback in this light too: today your body is rallying all its forces to have a good go at curing whatever is wrong. Once you have had a good moan, and laughed (hopefully) at the following page, set about helping your healing process with love and anything else you have found useful. Help your setback be very temporary.

Useless Things to Tell Yourself when you have a Setback

1. "This is only a little setback."
2. "Just think how much better you are than you were originally."

3. "Don't be upset about it. This isn't the end of the world."

4. "Don't feel bad about it."

5. "This serves you right for imagining you could ever be well again."

6. "You idiot, you should have known better than to have pushed that ten ton truck/bicycled to Africa/rescued that pensioner from drowning."

7. "If only you could love yourself enough, you would be well, why can't you love yourself, you useless lump of elephant turd?"

8. "After I tried *so* hard, body, how can you do this to me?"

9. "Ah well, there's always tomorrow....."

26

Conclusion

People usually fail when they are on the verge of success. So give as much care to the end as the beginning. Then there will be no failure.

(Lao Tsu: *Tao Te Ching.*)

What a wonderful journey to go through, and what a relief to come some, if not all of the way, out the other side. Or have we? Does our need for self-understanding, for love and attention ever stop? Does our potential to be ill ever diminish, or do we have to vigilantly follow the paths that encourage our health, not our sickness? If getting ill is a way of growing, are there any reasons to fear getting ill again? Can we continue to grow, and outgrow our need to be ill?

Being vigilant about our health does not mean avoiding that cream cake or chocolate or all night dance (unless we are sure it *will* make us sick) or anything else which gives us joy and excitement and makes life on this planet worth living, and feeling miserable in the process.

If a certain diet makes us healthy, we will want to keep to it, and if certain kinds of behaviour make us feel good we will want to follow those: vigilance means making sure we are keeping to the best for ourselves, not punishing ourselves by reducing our possible enjoyment.

Vigilance also means keeping a constant lookout for that

moment when we are about to slip from 11.30 to 12 o'clock and start the downward spiral.

Recently I watched a friend of mine work her way towards an illness. She began by being a little extra tired: she then slipped into "but I have to keep going because this and this needs doing" mode: she then began to feel everything relied on her keeping going, she then began to feel 'funny' every now and again, but ignored it, then she started to grit her teeth and struggle in order to keep going.... .

Luckily for my friend she was willing to realise what was happening, and let it all go. As soon as she started to feel unwell she took time off work, and spent time nurturing herself. She knew, after many years experience, not to push past this point, but to let everything go, and LISTEN TO HER OWN NEEDS. She realised that the "I've got to keep going everything relies on me" was in fact *part of illness setting in*, almost as if the body goes into spasm, or hypertension, and once it does that it is lost: either we STOP or we collapse.

Have you ever thought of catching yourself even before the unwell feelings set in? Have you ever thought of having a day (or three) in bed well? My son is hardly ever ill, and its possible that a little of the reason is because he's never connected a day at home getting love and attention, pottering about making things, hugging the fire, and feeling sleepy, with being ill. He can have a "day off" (as we call it) well, rather than spend several days off, ill and miserable. The advantage to spending the day in bed well is that you actually feel good enough to *enjoy* all those pleasures: like reading, making things, being looked after.

So before you go galloping off, fit and healthy, into the sunset, take some time to consider: what are the things about being ill that you like? What are the qualities illness provides that you need sometimes?

Is it: The quiet? The time to yourself, out of the main rushing river of your life? The lack of responsibility? The opportunity to be miserable? The chance to think about yourself and the meaning of your life, rather than be caught up in your daily routines? The attention? The feeling of being cared about and loved? The fact that people can't 'get at you' when you are down? The rest?

No doubt you can think of more things, some quite particular to you. If you write them down now, before you forget, maybe you will find time to provide them for yourself—regularly—whether you are ill or not, in the future.

Affirmations

An affirmation is not a way of 'jollying ourselves along', of trying to convince ourselves we feel good when really we feel awful. Nor is it an ideal—something distant and lofty we try to live up to. An affirmation, at its best, is a statement of fact. When we say, for example: "Every day in every way I am getting better and better" it is a statement of something we feel or know inside. It is said almost like a direction: "Turn left at the junction." "Get well today"—if we are clear we are simply describing something that 'is', we can be sure our affirmation will help.

Imagine an arrow with a string attached. I shoot the arrow into the dark (the unknown future) in a certain direction (health) and then follow the string to that place. If you can't believe in either the direction (health), or the arrow (your desire to be well), or the power of the string (the affirmation) then that is OK, but this approach may not be for you.

Different affirmations suit different people. For example, some people respond well to the idea of 'perfect health'—it excites them, captures their interest, and therefore motivates them. Others find 'perfect health' a difficult idea. I am, I must admit, among them. I have difficulty contemplating perfect health in an imperfect world, but this does not mean I can't aim for health—that is an improvement on what I now experience.

The principle behind affirmations is this: the power of

177

thought is immense. Thought can determine the shape of our life. If we replaced negative thoughts with positive ones, we can effect our lives accordingly.

For me an affirmation works best when it works to counter my own particular negative tendencies, rather than abstract ones. In other words it helps me not to fall into the dark pits I've dug for myself, to change certain beliefs through which I look at life. It also works best when it springs from a picture that I have of the direction I would like to go in: this picture is not something I decide on mentally, but instead 'comes out of me' when I do the exercise included in a minute.

However for those of you who wish it, I include a list of affirmations which you can try using to see if they feel 'good' or 'real' to you.

Affirmations can be written: for example, twenty-one times, three times a day. Or on a card or cards, and put up where they will be constantly read. They can also be memorised, and repeated mentally, especially at times when one feels oneself sinking into despair, lack of confidence, self-criticism.

"My body is vibrant, healthy and strong."

"Perfect health is the natural state of being."

"I will have a comfortable, restful sleep, and awaken filled with energy."

"My white cells circulate my body like light, destroying my illness, leaving me vibrant and healthy."

"I deserve health and strength."

"Every day in every way I am getting better and better."

Exercise to find personal affirmations.

Find a quiet, comfortable place to lie down. Begin by relaxing all the muscles of your body. Start with the toes; the feet; the ankles; the legs; the hips; the belly; the torso; the shoulders; the arms; the neck; the head; the face. Notice your breathing; allow your breathing to come and go, come and go without interference. Breathe right down your spine, picturing the air going right down the spine, circulating round the bottom of your pelvis, coming up the front of you, through your throat, and out. Breathe like this several times until you feel calm and relaxed.

Begin by picturing a circle of light surrounding your body from head to foot. Some people are better able to 'feel' rather than see a clear picture. Then picture yourself, some time in the future, well. What are you doing? How do you look? Use words in your mind which describe the image. These words will be useful for your affirmations.

It is possible that when you see it, you will find it difficult to believe in your picture. It may seem unclear, or a long way away. Ask yourself gently what gets in the way of your picture? Is there something you are afraid of? Is there something you doubt? Listen to your doubts and fears. Knowing these will help you create an affirmation that takes them into account.

Before you finish, tell yourself that you soon will be as well as your picture. Let the picture fade. Undo the circle around you (take it out the opposite way to the way you drew it) and come back to normal awareness.

Use the words you described your picture with, for example: vibrant, happy, dancing...in your affirmation. Remember to put it in the present tense. If we say "I will be well soon", we are not affirming our getting well now. We are putting it off to the future.

If certain negative feelings came up: fear we would die, fear that we didn't have the strength to get to the picture, for example, use the opposite thought in your affirmation.

If you have doubt: "I am confident in my healing abilities. I am now becoming well".

If you are afraid: "I trust in my body." Or "I know God is within me healing me." Stress belief, trust, being supported, being loved.

You may not believe it as you say it, but as you go on repeating it you will begin to feel more confident. An affirmation is a way of shaping your future by changing your present.

Visualisations

Visualisation is a very effective means of getting well—it has been used for healing all over the world for centuries. Visualisation is easiest to practise when we lie or sit in a relaxed manner and listen to someone's voices talking us through it. Mathew Manning has made an excellent tape "A Guide to Self-Healing". There are other excellent tapes on the market which you could find out about at your local health food/ alternative medicine shop.

Otherwise, if you have the facilities, you could record one of the following visualisations, and play it back to yourself—or simply have a friend with a nice soothing voice read it to you. Always read slowly and calmly.

Visualisation 1

This uses our medical knowledge about how the body heals itself: the primary factor in healing is our immune system which fights off infections, indeed all foreign bodies. Our white blood cells—and our T cells—go to the disturbed area, surround it, and heal it.

Begin by shutting your eyes and relaxing your body, starting with your toes. Let go of the tension in each toe on each foot, relaxing the arches of your feet, and your ankles. Let go of the tension in your legs, letting your knees relax, letting your thighs relax, letting go of all the tension in your pelvis, and buttocks. Allow your spine to relax, and soften, and all the muscles of your stomach to release, and the muscles of your back, and chest, and shoulders to relax. Allow your breath to move gently and deeply in your chest, relaxing your arms, and your wrists, and each finger right to the fingertips. Relax your neck all the way up to the top of your throat, relaxing your throat muscles, and allowing your tongue to spread out and rest on the floor of your mouth. Relax your head, and let all the muscles of your face, and jaw soften and let go. Allow your eyes to soften, and let your mind drop back inside you, so that you go deeper and deeper, and feel more and more relaxed. (*Pause*)

And as you move deeper and deeper into yourself, notice your breathing. Just follow your breath as it flows into your body, down into your lungs, moving your belly, lightly flowing down and then up and out. Follow your breath several times. (*Pause*)

Imagine your breath is making a circular movement. It comes into your body, down your spine, all the way down your spine to the bottom of your pelvis. Your breath circles round your pelvis and rises again at your pubic bone, coming up the front of your body, and out through your throat. Don't try to get a clear picture of this, if you don't have one, simply keep imagining the flow of air down your spine, around the bottom and up the front. (*Pause*)

Now imagine that as you breathe in the air you also breathe in light, and as the air comes into your lungs the light bubbles through your heart and into each blood cell which circulates around your body. So you can picture the light making the same journey as the air: down your spine, circulating your belly and pelvis, and up your front. (*Pause*)

This light which comes into your body on your breath, is a very healing light. Imagine it attaching itself to the white blood cells in your blood, so that the blood cells fill up with this light; so that the blood cells in your body are radiant with healing light. Follow your white blood cells—however you picture them, as dancers, or fighters, or cleaners, or any other image—as they move, shining with light, towards the area of your body which is in pain. (*Pause*)

Watch the white blood cells surrounding the area of pain, watch them moving into each dark crevice, comforting each angry red hurt. Feel their soothing radiance heal you. Keep feed yourself more and more light as you breathe slowly and deeply into your body, filling yourself with healing. (*Pause for a few minutes*)

Know that the natural healing power of your body is at work. Know that you are able to aid your own recovery. Know that you are able to care for yourself. Watch the white cells, and thank them for all they are doing. (*Pause*)

Now when you are ready you are going to return to ordinary consciousness, confident that you can leave your awareness of the white cells, because you know they are still working for you. As you travel again up your spine, on the outward breath, know that all is well in your body. When you are ready, open your eyes once more.

Visualisation 2

This takes us to a place in our imagination which gives us a feeling of serenity and peace and strength.

Find a comfortable position, making sure you are warm enough, and shut your eyes. Begin by relaxing your body, starting with your toes. Let go of the tension in each toe on each foot, relaxing the arches of your foot, and your ankles. Let go of the tension in your legs, letting your knees relax, letting your thighs relax, letting go of all the tension in your pelvis, and buttocks. Allow your spine to relax and soften, and all the muscles of your stomach to release, and the muscles of your back, and chest, and shoulders to relax. Breathe gently and deeply into your chest, relaxing your arms, and wrists, and each finger right to your fingertips. Relax your neck all the way up to the top of your throat, relaxing your throat muscles, and allowing your tongue to relax on to the floor of your mouth. Relax your head, and let all the muscles of your face, and jaw, soften and let go. Allow your eyes to soften and relax, and let your awareness drop back inside you, so that you go deeper and deeper, and feel more and more relaxed. (*Pause*)

Take a deep breath, imagining the air right down into your belly. Take several more deep breaths. (*Pause*)

Now you are ready to go deeper and deeper into warm relaxation. And now you can begin your journey. First of all imagine a ring of light surrounding your whole body. This light will protect you, and help you to feel relaxed, so imagine the light making a complete oval shape around you. (*Pause*)

And now imagine you can hear the sound of the sea some distance ahead of you. As you begin to walk in your mind's eye, you can see the sea. It is a beautiful blue colour, surrounded by soft golden sand. You can feel the warmth of the sun on your skin, making the surface of your skin glow, and expand in the warmth. You can smell the slight saltiness to the air, which floats on the gentle breeze.

As you walk slowly towards the sea, you can feel the softness of the sand underfoot. You may want to take your shoes off. You continue to walk, coming nearer to the vast sparkling blue of the ocean. As you see the ocean stretching out on either side of you, you feel yourself expand, and all the last remaining tension in your body seems to drop away.

You wander slowly along the sea's edge, enjoying the lyrical sound of the waves gently lapping on the shore. You may want to paddle in the sea, or simply watch the flecks of white foam as they froth on the golden sand. You are enjoying the warm sun, which is exactly the temperature you wish for. (*Pause*)

The blue of the sea seems to lift your spirit and bring a smile to your heart. You know this beach is perfectly safe, and the sea is wonderfully calm and reassuring. Spend some time just watching the rhythmic movement of the wavelets, and feeling the soothing quality of the water. (*Pause for several minutes*)

Now when you are ready you notice a clump of trees which are near the edge of the sand. The trees look protective and comforting.

Find one of the trees which seems most beautiful to you, and go up and touch its bark. Feel the solidity of its trunk, and imagine its roots going all the way down into the earth. Look up at its leaves, and allow the gentle green to touch your heart, and make you feel good.

Sit down now with your back against one tree so you can look out at the sand and sea, and rest your spine against the warm wood. As your spine relaxes against the wood allow yourself to be filled with the tree's serene strength. It is as if the tree is nurturing you, and filling you with strength. (*Pause several minutes*)

You are still warm, and as much sun as you wish reaches into the shade and touches your skin. You look out across the huge shining blue sapphire of the sea. A quiet serenity fills each part of your being. Nothing can worry you now. You are completely at ease. And you feel completely safe in a world which nurtures you, and fills you with joy. (*Pause for several minutes*)

This is your special place, and you can return here as often as you wish. Nothing can disturb you here. You are completely safe, and completely relaxed, enjoying the beauty which surrounds you. (*Pause*)

When you are ready you can choose to return to normal awareness. Become once again aware of your breathing, and of the feel of your body. Picture the circle of golden light which surrounds you, and undo the circle the opposite way to the way you drew it around you. Now you may open your eyes.

Visualisation 3

This takes us to a beautiful garden where we find a magical healing pond or stream.

Find a comfortable position, making sure you are warm enough, and shut your eyes. Begin by relaxing your body, starting with your toes. Let go of the tension in each toe on each foot, relaxing the arches of your foot, and your ankles. Let go of the tension in your legs, letting your knees relax, letting your thighs relax, letting go of all that tension in your pelvis and buttocks. Allow your spine to relax, and soften, and all the muscles of your stomach to release, and the muscles of your back, and chest and shoulders to relax. Breathe gently and deeply into your chest, relaxing your arms, and wrists, and each finger right down to your fingertips. Relax your neck all the way up to the top of your throat, relaxing your throat muscles, and allowing your tongue to relax onto the floor of your mouth. Relax your head, and let all the muscles of your face, and jaw, soften and let go. Allow your eyes to soften, and relax, and let your awareness drop back inside you, so that you go deeper and deeper, and feel more and more relaxed. (*Pause*)

Take a deep breath, taking the air right down into your belly. Take several more deep, calm breaths. (*Pause*)

Now you are ready to go deeper into relaxation, deeper and deeper. And now you can begin your journey. First of all imagine a ring of light surrounding your whole body. This light will protect you, and help you to feel relaxed, so imagine the light making a complete oval shape around you. (*Pause*)

And now imagine you are walking through a large green field in the middle of the country. The grass is short and makes soft swishing sounds under your feet. All around you the delightful green is dotted here and there with wild flowers. As you walk, you feel relaxed and free, like a child out to play. You look around you and for miles around you can see a beautiful view, which fills you with the sensation of spaciousness and comfort.

You walk for some time over the grass, enjoying the warm summer's day, and the fresh smell of everything around you. (*Pause*)

At the end of the field you come to a gate. Look at the gate carefully, and notice the intricate pattern marked on it. You can feel this gate leads to a secret, enchanting place, but you know that you may go in. Slowly you lift the latch and walk inside. You are now in a beautiful garden. As you walk along the path which leads through the garden you spend time looking at the bright splendour of the many flowers. Smell their delicate perfume. Bend and discover the tiny delicate buds hidden near the earth. Look up at the rich cascades of blossom.

Notice the multicoloured butterflies dancing from flower to flower. Listen to the sweet songs of the birds in the trees. This garden is your secret refuge, a place you can go to feel nurtured and uplifted. (*Pause for several minutes*)

Make your way on down the path, taking time to enjoy the calm loveliness of your surroundings. (*Pause*)

Suddenly you turn a corner and in front of you is a stretch of water. It may be a lovely still English pond. It may be a pool filled by a bubbling waterfall. Look at the water and notice its refreshing, peaceful quality. (*Pause*)

This is a healing pond or pool. The water has magic healing qualities which affect anything it touches. Stand at the edge of the pool, or pond, and take your clothes off. (*Pause*)

Walk slowly into the water: it is just the temperature to suit you, and it feels soft, and comforting. As you move deeper and deeper into the water, you can feel its vibrant healing filling your body. You feel good, and your muscles relax even more, until every last knot of tension is dissolved by the healing liquid. Continue moving into the water until it covers the place where your pain or illness is. (*Pause*)

As the water touches the place where you hurt, it is like a soothing balm, soothing away all pain. You can feel the energy of the water filling up the area and healing all the damage and distress. You can feel it stimulate and nurture your body's own natural healing. Allow the embrace of the water to gently comfort you, trust yourself to its soothing touch. (*Pause for several minutes*)

As the water supports and comforts you, you can feel how pure and caring it is. It holds you gently so that you are filled with the warmth of Love. Allow yourself to bask in this beautiful connection to the Universal Love: allow it to fill you right up, and chase away all your self doubts and self-criticisms. Know that you are perfect, and perfectly lovable right now. Know that the loving spirit of the water can go on and on pouring love into you, for there is no end to the Love, no end to the love, and you deserve as much as you need. (*Pause*)

Allow yourself to be filled right up to the brim with this still, gentle, joyful love. (*Pause for several minutes*)

The water will continue healing you, but you may decide now to play in it in some way: perhaps a swim, perhaps jumping and splashing. Take some time to enjoy being in the pond or pool, whether energetically or by simply floating lazily and watching the beauty of the garden all around you. (*Pause for several minutes*)

Now it is time to leave the pool or pond, but you can return to it any time you wish. This is your healing place, and it is here for you whenever you need it. (*Pause*)

At the edge of the pond or pool, dry yourself in the warm sunshine. You may want to get dressed again in your old clothes, or you may choose to put on the new clothes that are waiting for you. Notice their texture and colour. Notice how you feel as you put them on. (*Pause*)

When you leave the pond you walk a little way, and then find another gate back out of the garden into the field. Shut the gate behind you, so that your garden is safe, and walk out into the field again, experiencing the new sensation of health and strength inside you.

Know that you are getting better. Know that your body is busy healing you. Know that the health and strength and joy you now feel will always be within you. (*Pause*)

Know that you are a unique and fine person who fully deserves the love and healing you found in the pool or pond today. (*Pause*)

Undo the circle of light in the opposite direction to the one you drew it in. When you are ready, open your eyes.

Exercises for the Bedridden

1. Screw the face up, screw up the eyes, lips, and cheeks. Release. Repeat five times.
   Stretch the face, opening the jaw as wide as possible and sticking out the tongue. Repeat five times.

2. Turn the head to one side as far as you can. Turn it to the other side as far as you can. Repeat five times.

3. Roll the eyes in the head, in circular movement. First to the left, and then to the right. Repeat five times.

4. Open the hands as wide as you can, and then shut them as tight as you can. Repeat for as long as is comfortable.

5. Move the wrists in a circular motion, to the left and to the right. Repeat five times.

6. Move the toes of the foot. Wriggle them as much as possible. Move the feet backwards and forwards, and side to side. Repeat five times.

7. Squeeze the muscles of the pelvic floor five times. Release. Repeat five times.

8. Breath the air deeply into your body, imagining it down your spine, into your pelvis, filling your pelvic area. Push the air gently downwards. Hold. Release, imagining the air coming up the front of you, and allowing it out through the hips, with a puffing sound. Repeat 5 times.

Exercises for the Convalescent

Any simple set of movements will do which make you feel good. It is best to exercise to music, as the music helps your body move freely.

It is also better to do a little, once a day, than to knock yourself out doing too much, and not do it again. (of course!)

A suggested programme could be:

1. Shake your hands from the wrist. Shake your arms from the elbow. Shake the whole arm from the shoulders until it feels nice and loose.

2. Shake the foot from the ankle. Shake the leg from the knee. Shake the whole leg from the hip joint. Repeat for other leg.

3. Roll the head on one side, then to the other side. Move the head back, and then drop it forwards. Repeat gently in time with music.

4. Swing the arm in a circular movement, first forwards, then backwards in time with music.

5. Swing the body in a circular movement, first to one side then the other.

6. Push the arms forward, as hard as you can. Bring them back to your shoulders. Forward, back, quick and hard. Repeat.

7. Move legs apart. Bounce first on one leg and then on the other. Repeat.

8. If you feel up to it, jump a little in time with the music.

Further Reading

Health

Raw Energy: Leslie and Susannah Kenton (Century Hutchinson)

A lively and persuasive book about the value of raw foods. Even if you decide the diet is too extreme for you, there are some delicious recipes worth making use of.

Candida Albicans: Leon Chaittow (Thorsons)

If you suffer from tiredness, unexplained pelvic aches, a sense of unreality, nausea and your GP hasn't been able to help you—I advise you to seriously consider this diet. Some sufferers of ME claim to have benefited. Mr Chaittow explains carefully why and how it works.

Maximum Immunity: Michael A Weiner (Gateway Books)

An in-depth study of diseases of the immune system, and how to keep your immune system healthy.

General

The Bristol Programme: Penny Brohn (Century Hutchinson)

Penny Brohn's book is both inspiring and helpful, giving support and encouragement to anyone trying to recover from a serious illness (She had cancer), giving some useful approaches as well.

Finding a Way: Alex Howard (Gateway Books)

This is a therapy-made-simple book for those who find therapy a bit daunting, but who want to understand themselves better. Ill in bed for a bit—try this!

The Game of Life and How to Play it: Florence Scovel Shinn (Fowler)

My mother gave me this book when I was ill, and said if I could overcome the American enthusiasm I would find it was full of gems of wisdom. Sometimes—especially when you are ill—it is good to read someone who really believes enthusiastically. Florence believes in God, and the power of asking for what you need.

What you can feel you can Heal: John Grey (Heart Publishing, USA)

This introduction to therapy is made easy to read with the use of lots of amusing cartoons. If you can get hold of it, take a look.

Motherwit: Diane Mariechild (The Crossing Press, USA)

There are some beautiful psychic exercises in this book, written especially for women.

Open the Window: Joan Gibson (Gateway Books)

A very readable book written by someone who knows the problem of depression from the inside, giving practical ideas on how to combat it.

Body Learning: Michael Gelb (Aurum)

This book contains some lovely pictures as well as a most interesting outline of the Alexander Technique. If you can't get this I also recommend:

The Alexander Technique: Chris Stevens (Optima)

The Alexander Principle: Dr Wilfred Barlow (Arrow)

An Introduction to Spiritual Healing: Eileen Hertzberg (Thorsons)

This delightful and slim volume introduces the benefits of spiritual healing. Including practical questions such as "What does it feel like? Where do I go to get it?" as well as a fascinating background.

You can Heal your Life:
Heal your Body: Louise Hay (Eden Grove)

If you can beg, borrow or buy a copy of Louise Hay's books, or tapes, then do. She will inspire you to help yourself to health. Her voice on the tapes is sheer bliss: making you feel loved and cared for.

Tapes

There is nothing as soothing as listening to the voice of someone who inspires you with calm confidence and self love. It is a good way of guaranteeing yourself a time during the day when you will consciously set about being in a state of peace and healing. Apart from the Louise Hay tapes, I believe there is a good one by Shakti Gawain. There is also:

Energy Centres by Chris Jacobs

available by post from C Jacobs Energy Centres, 3 Alexander Rd, Penzance

Matthew Manning

has also produced a series of good tapes, ranging from "Reducing High Blood Pressure" to "Relief from Pain": Matthew Manning Centre, 39 Abbeygate St, Bury St. Edmunds, Suffolk, IP33 1LW.